LIFE AFTER
A HEART ATTACK

LIFE AFTER A HEART ATTACK
Social and Psychological Factors
Eight Years Later

Sydney H. Croog, Ph.D.

University of Connecticut Health Center
Farmington, Conn.

Sol Levine, Ph.D.

Boston University
Boston, Mass.

HUMAN SCIENCES PRESS, INC.
72 FIFTH AVENUE,
NEW YORK, N.Y. 10011

Printed in the United States of America
23456789 987654321

Library of Congress Cataloging in Publication Data

Croog, Sydney H.
  Life after a heart attack.

  Bibliography: p. 301
  Includes indexes.
    1. Heart—Infarction—Social aspects.   2. Heart—Infarction—Psychological
aspects.   3. Cardiacs—Rehabilitation.   I. Levine, Sol, 1922–.   II.
Title.   [DNLM: 1. Follow-up studies.   2. Myocardial infarction—
Psychology.   3. Myocardial infarction—Rehabilitation.   WG 300 C948L]
RC685.I6C77   362.1'961237   LC 81–6702
ISBN 0–89885–071–1   AACR2

To the memory of
John H. Knowles, M.D. and Leo G. Reeder, Ph.D.
in appreciation of their help in this study

and to
the heart patients and their families
whose generous participation made the entire project possible

CONTENTS

FOREWORD

Heroic efforts are often made to enable the heart attack victim to survive an initial or subsequent episode. The implication is often made that once recovery occurs the patient is "as good as new." We know that is not true since the recovered patient has lost some functioning myocardium and the fact that he or she had the attack in the first place is evidence of serious coronary atherosclerosis which, even without progression, may incite further ischemic episodes. On the other hand, many postmyocardial infarction patients can lead their usual lives with essentially normal life expectancy. The factors which affect these differences in outcome are numerous and important.

Physicians who take care of patients with coronary disease are familiar with the concerns of the patient and family members when recovery from the acute attack appears assured. Will I have another attack? Can I go back to work? How will this affect my life style and my relations with my family? What can I do to improve my chances of survival? These concerns and many other issues relating to "Life After a Heart Attack" are thoroughly and carefully studied in this book by Drs. Croog and Levine.

In a scientific 8-year follow-up of men who experienced an

9

initial myocardial infarction, the authors have obtained rich data regarding the social, psychological, and other factors which affect the lives of these men. Many of their findings are consistent with the experience of physicians who have had occasion to observe large numbers of such patients, especially if the relationship has been that of primary care physician. They have become well aware that the recovered myocardial infarct patient is still in the highest risk category for the reappearance of such an event and that many of these will be fatal.

Physicians will be pleased to find that many impressions they may have formed from personal observation are confirmed by Drs. Croog and Levine's unique and extensive study. One of the most significant of these is the finding that the medical assessment of health early after immediate recovery was one of the most important factors in predicting the health status of patients after many years. Those of us who have had occasion to engage in substandard insurance underwriting have long known that an uncomplicated recovery in a subject who could be pronounced quite healthy, except for the electrocardiographic marker of a previous myocardial infarction, carried a good prognosis. When combined with early return to work or resumption of usual activities, a particularly favorable prognosis could be made.

The authors have extended their observations well beyond these limited factors and have assessed the perceptions of the subjects as well as the many environmental factors which may affect the medical and social prognoses. They have also looked at the social, emotional, and financial problems which the post-myocardial infarct patient faces. In addition, the authors make a number of interesting policy recommendations. Altogether the findings are optimistic.

Physicians, nurses, social workers, and other health professionals can gain great confidence in counseling postmyocardial infarct patients from the material in this book. They can use the added knowledge to better advise their patients regarding any life style changes needed and to encourage positive attitudes in those who are unsure of the benefits of making any recommended changes.

One interesting finding which should make us all stop and think is the failure of more than a few of the subjects to utilize many of the various community services available to them and to rely almost exclusively on their physician relationship. The usual assumption has been that valuable services have been neglected and that greater efforts should be made to bring patients into closer contact with the service agencies. May the findings of this study not also suggest that we may have overvalued these services as seen from the patient's perspective? Further study of this subject seems highly warranted in view of the money and effort expended in providing the services.

I hope that physicians, nurses, social workers, and other health professionals will read this valuable book. Those who do will find themselves in a much better position to discuss the many problems facing heart attack victims and their families. The book will also be of immediate interest to heart patients and their families who may compare their own conditions and experiences with those in this study.

Thomas Royle Dawber, M.D., M.P.H.
Professor of Medicine
Boston University School of Medicine

ACKNOWLEDGMENTS

This report on heart patients is based on a follow-up study supported in part by Grant 10-P-57537 from the Social Security Administration (Health Services Use and Life Problems in Chronic Disease). The authors are grateful to the granting agency for its participation in the funding necessary to carry out the research.

This study is a reexamination of patients participating in an earlier project, "Social Factors in the Recovery of Heart Patients." That project was funded by U.S. Public Health Service Grant CD-00068, and it was located in the Department of Behavioral Sciences, Harvard School of Public Health. It was carried out in Boston as a 1-year prospective study of 345 male heart patients. Reports of findings from the earlier study appear in a series of articles and in the book by Croog and Levine, *The Heart Patient Recovers* (1977).

The earlier research in Boston provides the baseline and format for the current research. Data from the base-line study are joined with the new materials of the follow-up research, providing a basis for longitudinal analysis of a broad range of variables.

In the preparation of this report we therefore owe a double debt which we happily acknowledge. One is to all those who have made possible the completion of the long-term follow-up study, including its interviewing program, the analysis of data, and preparation of the manuscript. At the same time, we point out that the current report rests upon contributions of those who participated in the base-line study. Many of them already have been noted in *The Heart Patient Recovers*. Because of their important earlier contributions, many of the individuals who influenced the base-line study continue to help shape the current work.

In survey research of the size and duration of projects such as ours, the final products depend on the contributions of many people. As the total effort is cumulative, the efforts of each set of specialists and workers are critical to the integrity and accuracy of the total product. We wish to acknowledge here some contributions of our various colleagues and helpers in this joint effort.

Arnold Fieldman, M.D. served as Medical Consultant, offering important guidance in regard to a broad range of medical issues in administration of the project, data collection, and analysis. Warren M. Strauss, M.D. was Medical Director for the field study phase of the research in Boston, and he acted also as liaison with the physician group providing care for the patients. The study owes a special debt to both Drs. Fieldman and Strauss for their many informal contributions, as well as their formal participation in the medical management and physician liaison aspects.

The interviewing program for the project was carried out through the operation of a Field Office Unit, located at Boston University. Roberta K. Idelson, M.A. was both Field Office Coordinator and Research Associate, working in the Boston area. In addition to her effective administration of the interviewing program, she has an additional distinction as a tracer of respondents. After a period of over 7 years since previous contact, Ms. Idelson was able to locate or account for all of the 293 patients who had participated in the three-stage interview program of the base-line study.

The interviews were carried out by a core group of senior professionals. As they served with distinction in the base-line study, it was particularly fortuitous that they were available for this follow-up research. They were: Madeline Daniels, M.S.W., Gloria Long, M.S.W., Joanne Marks, M.S.W., John Trainor, M.S.W., and Samuel Pietropaolo, M.S.W.

Over the course of this research, the project employed a series of research assistants, and this report has benefited in many ways from the diligence, zeal, and motivation which they brought to their work. We refer particularly to Shifra Weinberg, Paul Gondek, Hope M. Cinquegrana, Nancy C. Prouser, Virginia Grudzien, Lawrence La Voie, Edward F. Fitzgerald, and Nancy P. Richards. All were located at the University of Connecticut Health Center.

Among the research assistants, several carried out extra tasks which had a distinctive imprint on the project, and they thus deserve further note. Our special thanks are due to: Edward Fitzgerald for supervision of the coding operation and for his work on the extensive coding instructions and on the system of data management; to Lawrence La Voie for his contributions to setting up the data file systems and for his guidance on issues involving statistical packages; and to Nancy P. Richards for her skilled performance of a wide variety of research tasks, including systems file management, data analysis, and editorial activities.

At the University of Connecticut Health Center the administrative management of the project was facilitated by Judy Klonoski and Marilyn Glenn. Edward Munster provided much patient and amiable guidance with our data management procedures and our use of the Univac 1106.

Along with this staff, we are grateful to the group of nine coders who labored in transforming interview responses into numerical data for computer analysis. This staff carried out the tasks with skill, good spirits, and understanding of the importance of their own work in building the research. They include: Regina Hibbeler, Kathryn Pearse, Ann Tait, Kay Rickles, Janet Smith, Virginia Crabtree, Virginia Grudzien, Greta Hopkins, and Nancy Woodworth.

Among the many persons who typed the various drafts of manuscript for this report, we particularly wish to thank the following for their high quality work: Marian Hughes, Edna Newmark, Marilyn Glenn, Elaine L. French, Rita Langevin, Laura E. Croog, Amy L. Croog, and Caroline Holmes.

From our colleagues and associates we have benefited from much consultation in the development of this work. Though the final decisions on matters are our own, we received much helpful advice on substantive issues, statistical procedures, and research design. For this, among others we thank S. Stephen Kegeles, Ph.D., Adrian Lund, Ph.D., Howard L. Bailit, D.M.D., Ph.D., Raymond Forer, Ph.D., and Jonathan Clive, Ph.D. We appreciate the valuable guidance and insights which we received over the course of this research from Henry P. Brehm, Ph.D., of the Social Security Administration.

In acknowledging the many contributions of others to this project, we must also note once again that the design and methods of the follow-up study continue to benefit from the good works of those who helped us shape the original base-line study. This follow-up work, after all, follows the basic format of that earlier study in many key respects. Thus, we wish to acknowledge again the efforts of some of those colleagues whose influence has continued here. These include our physician colleagues who were formerly the Medical Directors: H. Jack Geiger, M.D., David L. Rabin, M.D., and A. Philip Connelly, Jr., M.D. The statistical guidance provided by Robert Reed, Ph.D. and by Jacob Feldman, Ph.D. continued to be a useful touchstone over the years, supplemented by our current consultants and advisers. The contributions of Walter L. Johnson, Ph.D. to the interview schedules in the base-line study are reflected once again in the current work. These names are, of course, but a sampling of a long list of those participants in the earlier research whom we might mention once again.

Preparation of the final draft was aided considerably by comments and suggestions from C. David Jenkins, Ph.D., Jerome K. Myers, Ph.D., and William B. Kannel, M.D. We appreciate the editorial assistance of Ann Leibowitz in helping prepare the manuscript for publication.

Finally, our greatest debt, of course, is to the study population of men who so generously and freely participated in this research. We are also grateful to their physicians who completed questionnaires for us. One of the happiest aspects of this research for us personally was the opportunity to go back to the heart patients in the study group and to renew acquaintances. The meaning of this experience and our debt to these participants and their families cannot be expressed adequately in brief words here. We thank them at least in part through this report, hoping that in some way it will fulfill their motivations in sharing important aspects of their lives with us over the years.

The follow-up study, as well as the base-line study, have led to a series of publications on the heart patient population. Some of their findings are briefly touched upon at various points in chapters of this report. Readers wishing to pursue interests in other related publications based on this study population will find reference to them in the Bibliography.

Chapter 1

INTRODUCTION

How do heart patients fare years after their first coronary attack? How do they deal with their illness? What resources do they call on? Why do the processes of recovery and rehabilitation prove more difficult for some than others? Before experiencing their first heart attacks, the 345 men this study describes were pursuing their customary day-to-day activities, free of major illness.[1] It is what subsequently happened to them—changing their lives—that is the subject of this book.

This research was undertaken in an effort to examine in longitudinal perspective some of the social, psychological, and economic sequelae of heart disease. Our earlier book, *The Heart Patient Recovers* (1977), reported on the progress of the several hundred heart patients during the first year after their first myocardial infarction. This volume describes and analyzes long-term outcomes identified in a follow-up study 8 years after their original hospitalizations.

A prominent feature of our heart patient group is that, like the general population, it is getting along in years. At the time of the follow-up study, the median age of the patients was 59; nearly 20% were 65 or older. Living with chronic illness has been complicated for many of them by various physical, social, and psychological concomitants of aging. Though not originally conceived as a study of aging, many of the findings in this report may tell us a good deal about the heart patient in the older years.

In reporting on the long-term careers of the heart patients, we have focused on some of the most central aspects of their lives: health status, psychological status, work, family relationships, finances, use of services and cash benefit programs, and the doctor-patient relationship. Specifically, our principal aims have been:

1. To report on the morbidity and mortality experience of the study population over the course of 8 years.
2. To describe long-term life patterns and rehabilitation needs of the heart patients and to identify barriers to rehabilitation and recovery.
3. To describe use of health services, cash benefit programs, and other resources, with particular emphasis on the 12 months immediately preceding the follow-up interview at Year 8.
4. To examine possible associations between differing patterns of performance after 8 years and (a) variables identified in the base-line study, such as medical prognosis, physical activity level, mental health indicators, psychological self-ratings, marital consensus, and work history, and (b) variables derived from the 12 months preceding the follow-up study, such as patterns of illness, life crises, socioeconomic status, financial situation, and perception of illness.

Before describing our approach and orientation more fully, we will briefly review some aspects of the background, methods, and focus which helped shape this study.

THE RESEARCH CONTEXT OF THIS STUDY

While the major impact of communicable diseases in the United States has been declining in recent decades, problems of chronic disease have been gaining in magnitude. According to national studies, about 86% of the elderly have one or more

chronic health problems (Butler & Lewis, 1977). The consequences of chronic illnesses, in terms of physical disability and of
social, emotional, and economic cost, are vast and pervasive.

Among the chronic illnesses, diseases of the cardiovascular
system are the most prominent causes of disability and mortality.
In the United States diseases of the heart in particular account for
over one-third of total mortality each year. Among Americans
over 45, heart disease is the foremost cause of death. According
to National Health Survey data, diseases of the cardiovascular
system are the prime cause of disability (activity limitation).
Among males 65 and over, 200 per 1,000 reported heart conditions in 1974; the rate for the age group 45 to 64 was 97 per 1,000
persons (National Health Survey, 1974).

The problems of heart disease are complicated by the fact
that its acute phase typically occurs in the later years of life. While
often burdened by other physical disorders and disabilities as
well, heart patients may also be subject to emotional disorders
such as depression, anxiety, and hypochondria (Butler & Lewis,
1977). In some cases, social isolation, anomie, lack of access to
services, and economic deprivation add to the difficulty of coping
with this chronic illness and may complicate its burdens.

In themselves, the problems of an aging population are
massive and complex and their many ramifications of economic
loss, disability, and social and emotional costs have often been
brought to national attention and concern (Binstock & Shanas,
1976; Butler, 1975; Haber, 1970; Howards & Brehm, 1977;
Smith & Lilienfeld, 1971). When these issues are joined with
those of chronic illness, however, the problems are multiplied.
When a widely pervasive illness such as heart disease is involved,
the actual number of people affected is enlarged, for the consequences of heart disease involve not only the patient but family,
associates, work relationships, the health care system, agencies
providing cash benefit support, and many other elements of the
community.

*Longitudinal Data on Social and Psychological Factors in the Lives of
Older Heart Patients*

In recent years numerous intensive and large-scale investigations and clinical trials have been undertaken, testing methods of

treatment and clinical management of heart patients. Efforts to develop preventive services and programs are being given new emphasis. And the recent scientific literature contains numerous reports on return to work, morbidity, and mortality among heart patients.

Despite an increase in sophisticated research on the care of heart patients, social scientists and physicians have undertaken relatively few large-scale social and psychological studies of long-term adjustment to heart disease among older patients. Although research on the aftermath of cardiac disease and on rehabilitation has produced many significant contributions, much remains to be done. Some years ago, after critically appraising a series of prominent follow-up studies of myocardial infarction patients, Seigel and Loncin reached a conclusion which is still relevant: "there is still a considerable amount that is unknown and subject to disagreement with respect to the natural history of heart disease; . . . . the state of knowledge of what happens to an individual after an infarct is primitive" (Seigel & Loncin, 1969).

Similar observations can be made about the status of empirical data on the biological, psychological, and social aspects of aging. As Carp has noted, "stages [of life] past the attainment of maturity have received relatively little attention. . . . These later phases of life have yet to be discerned, separated, and described, let alone understood. The fragmentary knowledge about them makes impossible a balanced and comprehensive understanding of the course of human life" (Carp, 1972).

These quotations point up some key features of the research literature on heart disease and aging. The long-term social, psychological, and economic sequelae of heart disease have received less attention than the etiology and epidemiology of the illness. Consequently, we have little systematic empirical information concerning differential adaptation to cardiovascular disease by older patients (and their families), their rehabilitation needs, use of health services, and adjustments to disability and retirement. In particular, the influences of the broad framework of social, psychological, and situational components have rarely been studied in longitudinal perspective. Hence, we still know relatively little about variation within subsegments of older heart patients and its relation to socioeconomic status, age, educational background, and ethnic and racial origins (Atchley, 1972).

Some recent longitudinal studies have documented basic processes and problems in areas relevant to our concerns here. Prominent among them are the Framingham Heart Study (Dawber & Kannel, 1972; Kannel & Gordon, 1977), and the data bank established at Duke Medical School for long-term follow-up of the effects of medical management of heart disease (Rosati et al., 1975). The Health Insurance Plan in New York has been an important source of data on the course of heart disease (Shapiro et al., 1965). Other follow-up studies have focused on morbidity, mortality, and associated variables. Studies of social and psychological factors in the life careers of heart patients have been published by Finlayson and McEwen (1977) and by ourselves (Croog & Levine, 1977).

Taken together, however, these various efforts relate only in part to the work reported here. For example, medical studies of heart disease generally lack a major focus on social and psychological factors. Longitudinal studies of aging typically are not specifically concerned with heart disease and its consequences. Finally, the few social and psychological follow-up studies of heart disease usually deal primarily with middle-aged rather than older populations.

Work, Retirement, and the Heart Patient

In studies of chronic illness, some investigators have addressed such key issues as return to work, retirement, the meaning of work, and factors influencing the decision to retire (Binstock & Shanas, 1976; Blau, 1973; Riley & Foner, 1968; Sheppard, 1976). In fact, there has been an efflorescence of social science research linking these topics to larger theoretical issues involving life change, adaptation, and the life cycle. Various analytic frameworks have been proposed, such as those based on life stage theory, theories of social psychological adjustment, crisis theory, and disengagement theory. For example, Shanas examines two processes, *substitution* and *accommodation,* considering these in terms of their social process aspects and their implications both for individuals involved and for social structure (Shanas, 1972). Another approach to analysis of retirement is seen in the application of a life style typology or life career model, specifying differing patterns of retirement careers (Lowenthal, 1972). The concept of *disengagement,* while controversial, has stimulated much constructive debate (Cath, 1975; Cumming & Henry, 1961; Gordon, 1975).

In contrast to much detailed research emphasis on work and retirement as core issues in their own right, relatively little empirical research has been done on work and retirement in the lives of heart patients in particular. Perhaps the most prominent work-related focus in the literature on heart patients concerns issues of "return to work." This involves such questions as: Who returns? When? What can be done to facilitate it? How effective are various measures such as exercise programs in returning patients to work (Naughton & Hellerstein, 1973)?

Some recent studies have examined "return to work" and disability, following hospitalization, in relation to life adjustment and morale (Croog & Levine, 1977; Finlayson & McEwen, 1977; Garrity, 1973). Our own research, for example, found that being either a blue-collar or white-collar worker was an important element affecting the employment careers of middle-aged heart patients (Croog & Levine, 1977). Job satisfaction and work stress previous to the hospitalization have also been found to be important in affecting pattern of return to work (Blau, 1973; Garrity, 1973). However, we can still note that little research of a systematic, empirical nature has been done on the work adjustment or retirement experience of the older heart patient. Generalizing from younger age groups—or from the literature concerning aging—is a poor substitute for direct empirical data on the older heart patient.

The Aging Coronary Patient and Health Services

Among older heart patients, what is the pattern of use of services, and how does it vary within subpopulations with differing needs and social and demographic characteristics?

Our earlier, base-line study of male heart patients after hospitalization found minimal use of community health services, aside from physicians (Croog & Levine, 1977). A review of national trends by a Task Force of the Heart Institute does not contradict this finding on use of the hospital and the physician relative to other services in the community (Task Force on Cardiac Rehabilitation, 1974).

Age often serves as an important predictor of utilization of health services (Haber, 1968). Because older people have more chronic diseases, they tend to use more services (Andersen et al., 1970; Anderson & Andersen, 1972). People who are 65 and older are more likely than other age groups to be visited at home by physicians, and to respond to illness by visiting a physician (Andersen, 1968; Shanas, 1960). Hospital admission rates peak at ages 65 and older, and length of hospital stay increases steadily with age (Andersen et al., 1970). Patients in chronic disease hospitals are primarily the elderly (National Center for Health Statistics, 1970). People in the older age brackets spend more on hospital services than any other age group, and consumption of and expenditures for prescribed and over-the-counter drugs increase with age. Use of services has also been found to be related to such variables as awareness of facilities, life style, and characteristics of the community (Rosenzweig, 1975; Taietz, 1975).

However, these studies typically do not review use of health services by older heart patients in particular, a group which may have need for such services both because of heart disease and because of the array of other physical, social, and economic problems which confront an older population. A crucial related issue is the effect of such factors as economic situation, social class status, and degree of activism or depression on use of services by older heart patients.

Doctor-Patient Communication and Compliance

Two of the most pervasive problems clinical physicians face are ensuring adequate doctor-patient communication and compliance by the patient with the medical regimen (Becker & Maiman, 1975; Marston, 1970). In long-term chronic illness much responsibility for management falls to the patient himself, and involves self-care, taking medications consistently, and carrying out the medical regimen without continuing personal supervision by the physician. In the case of serious illness, such as heart disease, noncompliance with the regimen can have serious and even lethal consequences.

Doctor-patient communication is often more problematic with older patients. The usual barriers to communication may be accompanied by hearing loss and other handicaps (Ley & Spelman, 1965; Schwartz et al., 1962). Capacity to comply may be compromised by forgetfulness, confusion, anxiety, depression, and by such practical matters as cost, home situation, and physical limitations. Needless to say, not all older patients have such problems. Thus a persistent need exists for systematic detection of the patients most likely to have communication and compliance problems, and for designating special care, support, and supervision for these target populations.

Despite growing research interest in compliance and its concomitants, there has been relatively little empirical research on these problems in the aging chronically ill—and almost none on the older heart patient. Sackett and Haynes' (1976) recent review of 246 prominent studies of compliance with a medical regimen found virtually none focusing on the older heart patient. The same condition is evident in other major reviews of compliance research (Becker et al., 1977).

Many issues remain unresolved. For example, many studies have found no association between patient age and compliance; however, most of these studies concentrate on nonelderly age groups (Cuskey et al., 1971; Davis, 1968; Rae, 1972; Weintraub et al., 1973). Some researchers have postulated that noncompliance and medication errors are associated with extremes of age, since geriatric patients experience more isolation, forgetfulness, and self-neglect (Blackwell, 1973). Others suggest that such findings are oversimplifications (Schwartz et al., 1962), and that other variables might be responsible for apparent correlations between age and adherence (Kasl, 1975; Villafana & Mackbee, 1971).

Impressive efforts have recently been made to develop coherent theoretical models as means of explaining health-related behavior relating to compliance. One example is the Health Belief Model (Kirscht, 1974; Rosenstock, 1974). However, the degree to which elements of threat, susceptibility, belief in the power of prevention, and other components of this model hold for the older heart patient has yet to be empirically determined.

Our earlier work on predominantly middle-aged heart patients produced mixed findings with regard to associations between compliance with the medical regimen and social and psychological variables (Croog & Levine, 1977). It may be that the special features of the disease—its life-threatening nature, its unpredictability, and the memory of great pain—outweigh the effects of other variables, at least in a middle-aged population. Croog and Richards (1977) found high compliance with medical advice to stop smoking among the heart patients. However, there was virtually no change in smoking habits among their wives. Such data suggest that components of the Health Belief Model, if they are operative, have differential effect on male heart patients and women who are not ill. How these factors affect compliance on the part of the older patient will be explored in Chapter 5, as we return to the same patients 8 years later.

Aging, Emotional Status, and Heart Disease

The statistical relationship between mental health problems and advanced age has been well documented in psychiatric epidemiological surveys, although estimates vary regarding the degree of association (Langner & Michael, 1963; Leighton, 1959). It has been estimated that from one-fifth to two-thirds of Americans aged 65 and over have some degree of psychiatric impairment (Epstein, 1976; Fann & Wheless, 1975). Nearly 90% of a San Francisco geriatric screening clinic's respondents were reported to require psychiatric care (a finding consistent with the purposes of the agency); of particular relevance here is that a high proportion were also diagnosed as physically impaired (Simon et al., 1970).

What becomes of elderly people suffering from depression, anxiety, and other emotional impairments complicated by the presence of life-threatening illness? How do emotional responses to heart disease compound the problems of rehabilitation and recovery? Among primarily middle-aged heart patients, the phenomena of anxiety, denial, and depression have been examined more in terms of their development and progression than their long-term effects (Bruhn et al., 1971; Croog, Shapiro & Levine, 1971; Hackett & Cassem, 1973). Indeed, most research on the emotional aspects of heart disease is concerned primarily with etiology rather than with the posthospital sequelae of the illness (Jenkins, 1976).

Although there are complex interrelationships between the

course of heart disease and changes in emotional status, they have not often been systematically examined in tandem, aside from studies focused on small clinical series. The association between the two issues raises further questions about the possible influences of a heart patient's troubled emotional status upon such other areas of life as work, retirement, and family. Concomitantly, we still have much to learn about how heart patients from different social levels manage the loneliness, despair, and uncertainty that sometimes characterize old age.

Family and Social Networks: The Aging Heart Patient

Many aspects of family life and of other elements in the social network interact with how the aging heart patient deals with this illness. Some new and relevant materials have been emerging in research on the family life of older persons, on their home or institutional life situations, and on their participation in social networks (Blau, 1973; Solon et al., 1977; Sussman, 1976). But in regard to the older, chronically ill—and within the older coronary disease population in particular—many issues remain unresolved both in regard to main patterns, and in regard to specific subgroups (Croog, 1970; Task Force on Cardiac Rehabilitation, 1974).

For example, questions about the role of the family in modern industrial society have led to crossnational research on the nature of kinship networks and on ways in which kin interact and provide mutual support (Kaplan et al., 1977; Sussman, 1959, 1976). Studies have shown there is far more interaction and support than had been commonly supposed by theorists holding that the extended family is declining radically in importance. Yet the empirical research on interaction and support shows variation by socioeconomic level, by geographic area, by cultural origin, and a series of other variables. Given this mixed pattern of reports on the "family" as a generic type, it is not surprising that few data are available on the older heart patient in particular in regard to matters of interaction and support.

Our own research on 345 middle-aged heart patients found patterns of support and aid to be associated with the age of the patient, as well as with his degree of social integration and general level of social participation (Croog et al., 1972). Variation by social level, such as that reported in studies of nonpatient groups, was not evident in the data. One conspicuous finding was the high degree of support and aid from non-kin persons such as friends and neighbors, who tended to function in important ways as quasi-family for the heart patients. One question is whether these patterns may also be found among aging heart patients—whose family situations are quite distinctive in many ways from those of younger men.

Another type of question relates to the emotional impact of chronic illness upon the home, upon family relations and, in turn, upon the patient. Within both older and younger age groups the impact of illness varies (Skelton & Dominian, 1973), although the correlates and antecedents of response by family members to a seriously ill person are not yet well documented. In our own research, some notion of emotional tone in the home is implied by the finding that in over one-third of marriages of 300 heart patients, one or both partners blamed conflict with the wife as a cause of the illness (Croog, 1975). How the character of family life and the degree of interpersonal tension affect the course of adaptation to illness by the older patient is one of the areas which deserves further exploration.

Much of the recovery and rehabilitation of the long-term coronary patient occurs in the home after discharge from hospital (Finlayson & McEwen, 1977). This has important implications with regard to the capacity of physicians to make constructive use of the family itself in the therapeutic regimen. However, the limited empirical data on aging heart patients and the roles of their families in coping with illness often stands as a handicap to effective care and community program planning with this population (Sussman, 1976).

Quality of Life Among Aging Heart Patients

What is the quality of life for the aging person after a heart attack? In older individuals who must deal with the prospect of approaching death, personal loss, marked changes in family and in social relationships, and with other problems of their age group, what are the consequences of the additional burdens of a chronic disease which unpredictably and instantly can be lethal?

Here, as in some other areas of heart patient research we

have surveyed, there are few empirical studies which examine this important issue and which systematically describe significant variations within various subgroups of older heart patients. In the field of aging research, however, the particular dimensions of quality of life and life satisfaction have received comparatively greater attention, both as empirical phenomena in themselves (Spreitzer & Snyder, 1974; Streib, 1956) and as an integral part of theoretical schemes explaining the aging process (Carp, 1972; Cumming & Henry, 1961). Research findings in the literature on life satisfaction and aging (Butler & Lewis, 1977; Lowenthal et al., 1975; Maas & Kuypers, 1974) show that life satisfaction and high morale in earlier stages of life seem to be associated with these same features years later. In a study of aged persons, using path analysis techniques Medley found health to be less important as a predictor of life satisfaction than other studies have posited. Other areas of life, particularly family relationships and standard of living, were most closely related to life satisfaction (Medley, 1976).

This research and other work serve to point up the continuing condition: inadequate data on variation within subgroups as it relates to the life satisfaction and quality of life variables. As Medley remarks, "Much of the earlier and some present research presents a monolithic picture of life among older persons. . . . The data reported here support the need to study differences within older age groups. . . . Generalizations drawn from simple age group comparisons are at best highly tenuous and overlook the tremendous variations within the age groups" (1976). It seems evident that this comment may be valid for studies of older heart patients as well.

Aging as a Characteristic of the Study Population and Age as an Analytic Variable

In this book, we will be looking at issues involving age in two ways. First, we are concerned with age as a characteristic of the study population as a whole, describing situations and problems of men moving along into their elder years. Second, we will also examine age as a specific independent variable, focusing on its relationship to other variables in this report. In using the age variable for these analytic purposes, we must note that the age range of the study population refers to a particular span of years, based on the initial study design.

In Sum

These are some of the issues and contingencies which have influenced the formulation of this research. At this point in the development of knowledge concerning heart disease and use of resources and services, the need for empirical research with a broad integrated approach is clear. We need to examine the differing life career patterns of the older heart patients and the social, psychological, and economic factors that influence their responses to the problems of aging and of heart disease. These broad issues also raise questions about doctor-patient communication and compliance among the elderly, disability and its correlates, and problems of work, retirement, and finances. We need to fill large gaps of information in regard to variation in pattern, particularly those which relate to differences in socioeconomic status, age level, health level, and other social and demographic characteristics. Many of the important issues concerning the life careers of heart patients can perhaps best be addressed by longitudinal studies, which permit us to follow patients over a period of years.

Methods and Orientation

This report is based on data collected over an 8-year period, in two phases: (1) a base-line study covering 1 year in the life of each patient, and (2) a follow-up study approximately 7 years later. A complete description of our methodological approach appears as Appendix A. The procedures and orientation of the base-line study are reported in detail in *The Heart Patient Recovers* (1977).

The original base-line study population consisted of 345 Caucasian males, previously without major illness, who had recently suffered a first myocardial infarction and experienced a noncomplicated clinical course of hospitalization. Thus this study reports on a relatively "pure" heart patient population, free of the confounding effects of additional illnesses and complications. All were between the ages of 30 and 60, and resided in the areas of greater Boston or Worcester, Massachusetts. All were screened by project physicians to ensure that they met the strict health status criteria for inclusion in the study.

Data were collected in a four-stage interview program utilizing survey research instruments and specially trained interviewers.* The first interview with the patient (Week 3) took place shortly before discharge from the hospital. On average, they occurred 18 days after admission for the myocardial infarction. Subsequent interviews took place 1 month after discharge (Week 7), 1 year after the initial admission to the hospital (Year 1), and approximately 8 years after the initial hospitalization (Year 8). Over the course of 8 years the original study population was reduced to a core population of 205 patients, primarily due to death.[2]

The first interview, designed to engage the patients in the study and to elicit demographic information, was relatively brief. Patients were asked about early symptoms, how they came to be under care, and their future plans. The subsequent interviews were longer and more detailed, covering many aspects of the patient's life, including compliance with medical advice, work, financial situation, family relationships, and social participation. For purposes of comparison and assessment of change over the course of the illness, the last three interviews had essentially the same formats (see Table 1-1).

At the time of the second and third interviews, the patient's wife or a close relative was interviewed separately. It was not possible to interview wives in the follow-up study at Year 8.

Data on the patients' health status, functional capacity, car-

*Throughout this volume, the terms *Week 3, Week 7, Year 1, and Year 8* will be used to designate the four sets of interviews and the periods when they occurred. This system of labeling differs from the one we used in our first book (Croog & Levine, 1977). In that work the symbols *T1, T2, and T3* were employed to indicate the first three patient interviews at Week 3, Week 7, and Year 1, respectively.

Table 1-1. Time Schedule and Outline of Topic Areas

Heart Patient Study Interview Program

	Patient Interview	*Spouse or Relative Interview*	*Physician Questionnaire*
Week 3	*N = 348*		
	Pre-Illness Health and Symptoms Denial Work Status and Plans Family Structure Physician Discussion of Illness		
Week 7	*Patient Interview* *N = 345*	*Spouse or Relative Interview* *N = 306*	*Physician Questionnaire* *N = 324*

	Use of Physician
	  and other Services
	Work
	Finances
	Personal and Social
	  Habits
	Perceived Etiology
	  of Heart Attack
	Family and Marriage
	Religion
	Pre-Illness Stress
	  and Personality
	Physician Advice
	  and Compliance
		Patient Care
		Perceived Etiology
		  of Heart Attack
		Patient Health
		  and Progress
		Use of Services
		Work
		Family and Marriage
		Religion
		Personality and
		  Stress
			Areas of Advice
			Therapy
			Prediction of
			  Patient Limita-
			  tions at 1 Year

Year 1	*Patient Interview* *N = 293*	*Spouse or Relative Interview* *N = 247*	*Physician Questionnaire* *N = 269*

	Use of Physician
	  and Other Services
	Work
	Finances
	Personal and Social
	  Habits
	Perceived Etiology
	  of Heart Attack
	Family and Marriage
	Religion
	Personality (Self
	  and Spouse)
	Physician Advice
	  and Compliance
	Rating of Health
	  and Symptoms
	Sources of Help
		Patient Care
		Perceived Etiology
		  of Heart Attack
		Patient Health
		  and Progress
		Use of Services
		Work
		Family and Marriage
		Religion
		Personality and
		  Stress (Self and
		  Spouse)
			Patient Status
			  at 1 Year
			Appointments
			Advice, Therapy
			  and Medication
			Severity of
			  Infarction
			Patient Adjust-
			  ment

31

Table 1-1.   (Continued)

Year 8	*Patient Interview* *N = 205*	*Spouse or Relative Interview* ――	*Physician Questionnaire* *N = 148*
	Use of Physician and Other Services Work Finances Personal and Social Habits Perceived Etiology of Heart Attack Family and Marriage Religion Personality and Stress Physician Advice and Compliance Rating of Health and Symptoms Sources of Help Hospitalization History Receipt of Health Assistance Benefits		Patient Cardiac Status Patient Cardiac Prognosis Total Health Status of Patient Date of Last Visit Medical Problems Which Handicap Patient

diac prognosis, and compliance with physicians' instructions were obtained from their physicians by questionnaires. These were completed at the time of the Week 7, Year 1, and Year 8 interviews.

A Framework for Analysis: The Patient's Armory of Resources

In order to realize the principal aims of the study, we have had to collect and assemble a wide array of data. In gathering, organizing, and analyzing these myriad data, we have found it useful to employ as one frame of reference the concept of an *armory of resources* or set of supports, which the individual may draw upon to cope with problems. This armory may be visualized as consisting of the total array of available social, psychological, and institutional and community resources. Its scope may be seen in terms of three levels: (1) *purely individual* resources, such as personality defense mechanisms and physical status; (2) resources that derive from *larger social or institutional structures,* such as family, church, work, and friendship networks; and (3) community resources which consist of such *formal organizational systems* as hospitals, rehabilitation clinics, the physician-medical care network, and federal and local agencies that provide income maintenance programs and other services. The armory of resources is not a new concept and it appears in various forms in the literature. We are attempting to build on previous knowledge by employing this concept as a means of describing in an integrated way those elements which may be associated with differential types of outcome in the case of a serious chronic disease.

As part of our analysis, we chose first to classify and delineate the types of resources available to the heart patients in the study. These were arrayed in two categories, premorbid and postmorbid.

Premorbid resources, as examined in this study, consist of those that existed prior to the first myocardial infarction. Data on the resources are drawn from the base-line study, particularly the first and second interviews. Premorbid resources include personality defense mechanisms; family cohesion; integrated social participation; availability of medical and institutional services, insurance, cash benefits, and pensions; financial competence; and flexibility on the job.

Postmorbid resources examined in this report can be differentiated on the basis of their placement in two time periods. The first and more important set consists of resources available or present during the *1-year period* preceding the interview at Year 8. Some of these resources include indices of constructive family response to the illness; use of medical services; supportive activities on the part of key individuals such as the patient's employer, physician, and children; adaptability of life plans; and such formal supportive services as cardiac clinics, public and private cash benefit programs, and other income supports. The second set is concerned with the total period following the initial myocardial infarction, consisting of approximately an *8-year period.* Because of the extended period of time involved, interpretation of data concerning these resources must be carried out with special caution. In employing measures of these resources, we refer mainly to general patterning, e.g., the continuing existence of a marriage, maintenance of work status, and use of community health care facilities.

Our second task has been to describe the resources available to and employed by different segments of the population, including those of varying social classes and ethnic or religious groups. Our effort has been to determine ways in which social characteristics are related to differential use of particular social, psychological, and institutional resources.

Third, we have examined various types of resources in relation to indices of outcome at Year 8. This was done both for the study population as a whole and for subcategories of patients, classified according to age, social status, an index of functional capacity, and other variables.

In order to explore and compare possible relationships between use of resources and both short-term and long-term outcomes, we have also examined differential use of resources at two points in time, Year 1 and Year 8, 7 years apart.

In sum, we adopted this multifaceted approach in order to facilitate (1) delineation of the types of resources employed by various subsegments of the heart patient population, and (2) description of possible relationships between differential use of resources and differential outcomes within these subpopulations. We hoped such an approach would enable us to appraise—at least in a preliminary way—the relative importance of the resources in the "armory" of individuals and the use of these resources in coping with life events.

FORMAT OF THIS REPORT

Using the methods and approaches described above, we have collected a broad range of social and psychological data on a relatively "pure" group of heart patients—all initially free of the confounding effects of other illness. As our review of the literature indicates, there have been few long-term, prospective studies similar to ours concerning the social and psychological sequelae of illness. The substantial expenses—in terms of time, money, and human resources—of such studies make it unlikely there will be many in the near future.

In presenting our findings we have pursued a relatively conservative policy. As the level of our data is predominantly nominal or ordinal, we have chosen to rely mainly on nonparametric tests as our statistical tools. We have tried to orient the analysis as closely as possible to the data, in order to prevent artifacts of complex statistical methods from inordinately intruding.[3]

It has been one of our principal aims to document and record our findings as part of the larger natural history of chronic heart disease. We hope this approach will facilitate future comparative analysis of these data with other study populations in similar prospective longitudinal research.

In the next chapter we discuss the morbidity and mortality experience of the study population over approximately 8 years. Subsequent chapters present data concerning primary areas of resources and supports in recovery and rehabilitation. Thus we turn in Chapter 3 to factors in the work and employment situations of the patients. Chapter 3 also examines the impact of the illness on personal finances, and the costs of the illness itself. Chapter 4 presents data on use of services and cash benefit programs. Chapter 5 reports on the doctor-patient relationship, with particular attention to compliance with the medical regimen.

Chapter 6 considers the role of the family in the long-term life careers of the heart patients and the impact of the illness on the family. Chapter 7 is concerned with aspects of psychological and emotional status of the patients. Chapter 8 presents an overview of variables related to differing patterns of outcome at the conclusion of the 8-year period. In Chapter 9, we summarize the findings and consider some of their implications for planning of health services, medical care, and understanding of the long-term process of coping with chronic illness.

NOTES

1. This research began with a study population of 348 men, all of whom were interviewed in the hospital shortly before discharge following treatment for their first myocardial infarction. In tracing mortality we refer to this number throughout the book. Three men died before they could be seen for a second interview at home.

Hence, for discussions of social and psychological factors, our core population numbers 345 men.

2.   See Chapter 2 and Appendix A for information on changes in the study population size and associated factors.

3.   The chi-square test and the gamma correlation are our principal statistical tools. Level of significance has been set at .05.

Since this is an exploratory study, we consider it desirable to report findings that are in the direction of significance but do not meet the formal criteria. Hence, we also report on findings at the .10 and .20 levels if they form a consistent pattern that might deserve future follow-up by other investigators. Such results are noted in the text as being in the direction of significance and suggestive of trends.

Chapter 2

MORBIDITY, HOSPITALIZATION, AND MORTALITY

In many respects our initial study population constituted an "elite" group among heart patients. They were men who had been in apparent good health before their first heart attack, i.e., without recognized major or significant illness. Their hospitalization for the first myocardial infarction had a noncomplicated course. Before their first heart attack they were fully involved in their occupational careers, and most were in the prime years of middle-age between 40 and 60.

What happened to the health of these men over the 8 years following their first heart attack? Which of their preexisting characteristics—that is, which antecedent variables—helped predict their long-term health outcomes? And to what extent did their previous health status, an important part of the "armory of resources," affect long-term outcome in terms of morbidity and mortality?

As we reported in our earlier study (1977), during the year following their first heart attack, approximately 5% of the original core group of 345 patients died. About 20% were rehospitalized, mostly for heart disease. According to their physicians, approximately 25% developed further significant symptoms of coronary disease. Thus nearly half the population continued to have serious problems with heart disease during that first year, although the death rate was relatively low.

We shall see that the subsequent medical histories of the patients, while favorable in many respects, testify to the continuing serious course of cardiovascular disease. They also show a general pattern of relatively minimal impairment in the performance of daily activities.

In this chapter we shall employ two methods of reporting on mortality and morbidity for the 8-year term of the study. One is a simple accounting, covering the entire period from the first interview to the last. The duration of this period varies slightly from patient to patient, depending on the various exigencies affecting scheduling of interviews to coincide with an 8-year anniversary of initial hospitalization. The second standardized approach is to examine the mortality and morbidity data for a uniform surveillance period, extending from initial entry into the study until a point 8.0 years thereafter. (For further information on methods, see Note 1 at the end of this chapter.)

The Total Interview Period: Week 3 to Year 8

During the total study period of 8 years after the first heart attack, a considerable proportion of the patients experienced health problems requiring hospitalization, and over one-fourth died. As Table 2–1 shows, the major health risk to the patients was their coronary artery disease.

Of the 95 men who died during this period, most (86%) died of heart disease. Within this latter group the predominant cause of death was myocardial infarction ($N = 67$), as identified by death certificates and/or physician reports. The next most prominent cause of death was cancer (eight men).

Another 143 men were rehospitalized one or more times and survived. Of these men, 55% were rehospitalized for heart disease at least once, and some of these were hospitalized at other times for other illnesses as well. Other than heart disease, the main reasons for hospitalizations were cancer, diseases of the gastrointestinal tract, and conditions of the musculoskeletal system.

Table 2-1. Mortality and Rehospitalization Between
First Hospital Admission and Year 8 Interview

Outcome	Number	Percent	Combined Percent
Deceased			
Heart disease	82	23.6 ⟩	
Other causes	12	3.4 ⟩	27.3
No information on cause of death	1	.3 ⟩	
Living, Rehospitalized One or More Times			
Heart disease*	79	22.7 ⟩	
Other causes	64	18.4 ⟩	41.1
Living, Not Rehospitalized	85	24.4	24.4
Living, Incomplete Information on Rehospitalization	24	6.9	6.9
No Information on Mortality Status	1	.3	.3
Total†	348	100.0	100.0

*In the case of rehospitalizations for heart disease as well
as for non-heart causes, patients are classified in terms
of primary category of interest here, "heart disease."

†The total population of 348 includes the core population of
345 at Week 7 and 3 patients who died between Week 3 and
Week 7.

In evaluating these findings on illness over the 8-year period,
it should be kept in mind that a significant degree of illness is
characteristic of a population of aging men. In one single recent
year, for example, 20% of American men aged 55 to 59 were
hospitalized in short-term hospitals (USDHEW, 1978).

Table 2–2 shows mortality and rehospitalization rates for the

Table 2-2. Mortality and Rehospitalization
Between Year 1 and Year 8 Interviews

Outcome	Number	Percent	Combined Percent
Deceased			
Heart disease	60	20.5	23.6
Other causes	9	3.1	
Living, Rehospitalized One or More Times			
Heart disease[*]	74	25.3	47.1
Other causes	64	21.8	
Living, Not Rehospitalized	82	28.0	28.0
Living, Incomplete Information on Rehospitalization	3	1.0	1.0
No Information on Mortality Status	1	.3	.3
Total[†]	293	100.0	100.0

[*] In the case of rehospitalizations for heart disease as well as for non-heart causes, patients are classified in terms of primary category of interest here, "heart disease."

[†] The population of 293 includes all patients who participated in the Year 1 interview.

interval between the Year 1 and the Year 8 interviews, the period which is the primary focus for this book. As may be seen, the proportions in Tables 2–1 and 2–2 are essentially similar. We present these data as part of our documentation of the experience of the heart patient group during the follow-up period succeeding our first study. Readers interested in detailed findings on mortality and morbidity during the first year alone are

referred to our earlier report, *The Heart Patient Recovers* (1977).
What do these data tell us about the total pattern of illness experienced by the patients? First, most men were severely ill at some time during the full study period, as evidenced by the data on deaths and rehospitalizations. We know that not more than an approximate 30% survived and were sufficiently healthy to be able to remain out of the hospital. Second, a well-known pattern of continued risk of recurrence of acute episodes of heart disease is evident, along with evidence of high mortality from heart disease. For example, among those men who died and among the survivors who had been rehospitalized at least once, two-thirds had a diagnosis of heart disease as a cause of death and/or a rehospitalization.

THE UNIFORM SURVEILLANCE PERIOD: FIRST INTERVIEW TO 8.0 YEARS

Turning to the standardized period covering the first 8 years (e.g., 8.0 years) we can see that the rate of death from heart disease was relatively constant (see Table 2–3).[1] Deaths from heart disease as a percentage of survivors ranged between 5.0 and 6.7% at each 2-year interval. Although the number of intervals in the table is small, it appears that after an initial decline, the death rate rose to its highest point during the 6.1 to 8.0 year period.

As there were relatively few deaths from causes other than heart disease during the 8 years, the combined data on deaths from all causes show rates essentially similar to those for heart disease deaths alone.

How do the 8-year findings from this study of heart patients relate to reports from longitudinal studies by others on survival and on recurrence of heart attacks? Direct comparisons between reports by various investigators cannot usually be made because of differences in methods, characteristics of patient populations, sample size, and other factors (Kannel, Sorlie, & McNamara, 1979). Further, in attempting any comparisons, we must note that our surveillance period begins after discharge from the hospital, and our data therefore are distinctive from those in studies which include mortality of the first days after infarction in their estimates of survival.

Nevertheless, some previous research by others can provide

Table 2-3.   Deaths in the Study Population as
of 8.0 Years After the First Heart Attack.   N = 345.

Years Since First Admission to Hospital	Death Rates: From Heart Disease			Death Rates: From All Causes [§]	
	Number of Deaths	Rate as a Percentage of Base Population[*]	Rate per 100 Patients in Surviving Cohort[‡]	Number of Deaths	Rate as a Percentage of Base Population
0.0–2.0	21	6.1	6.1	23	6.7
2.1–4.0	16	4.6	5.0	17	4.9
4.1–6.0	17	4.9	5.6	20	5.8
6.1–8.0	19	5.5	6.7	24	7.0
8.1–8.9[†]	9	–	–	11	–
Total	82			95	

[*]Base N = original total population of 348, less 2 men who withdrew from the study at Year 1 for whom we have no information on date of death, and 1 man whose mortality status is unknown.

[†]Data for interval are incomplete because of no information on the fate of the men after their Year 8 interview.   See Note 1.

[‡]The surviving cohort for each interval is computed as the base population of 345 minus the total number of deaths from all causes up to the beginning of that time interval.

[§] Death rate from all causes, including heart disease.

a general perspective on our data. For example, among males an average mortality rate of 5% from myocardial infarction was found in the Framingham Heart Study over a follow-up period ranging from Year 1 to Year 6 following first infarction (Kannel, Sorlie, & McNamara, 1979). In a study of heart disease patients in the Health Insurance Plan of Greater New York, researchers report that among men who survived their first heart attack for 1 month, 22% died of heart disease within 5 years (Weinblatt, Shapiro, & Frank, 1973). High mortality from heart disease rather than from other causes among patients with a first myocardial infarction has been well documented in numerous studies. Despite the noncomparability of methods, these findings from other studies imply that the long-term survival and mortality experience of the heart patients in this study were not unique to this group.

AGE AT ENTRY INTO THE STUDY AND SEVERE CARDIAC EVENTS: DEATHS AND REHOSPITALIZATIONS WITH SURVIVAL

Although age, mortality, and morbidity are prominently linked in the case of numerous illnesses, our data do not show a clear association in the case of this population of men with heart disease over the course of 8 years. As Table 2–4 shows, no linear trend is apparent with regard to age and death from heart disease during the full study period (column A). The same point can be made with regard to the incidence of a "severe recurrence," death, or at least one rehospitalization for heart disease with survival (see Note 5).

In evaluating these findings on age, we must keep in mind that they refer to a study population with a specified age range, as required by the study design. We present these materials in order to document characteristics of the study population over time. These data cannot be construed as questioning or contradicting the well-known associations between coronary morbidity/mortality, and the full range of age groups in the population as a whole.

HEALTH STATUS AND REHOSPITALIZATION HISTORY AT YEAR 8

Eight years after they entered the hospital for a first heart attack, what was the health status of the men in the surviving study population? At the time of their Year 8 interview, the patients were now 59 years old, on average. In contrast to their excellent health history prior to entry into this study, all now had an extended experience of living with heart disease. Some had other serious ailments as well. Among these survivors, as we saw earlier, a high proportion had been so seriously ill as to require rehospitalization for treatment of coronary or other health problems.

In the next pages we present data on the construct, *health*

Table 2-4. "Severe Recurrence" of Heart Disease From Week 3 to 8.0 Years. By Age at First Hospital Admission

Age at First Hospital Admission (N)	A Deceased Due to Heart Disease	B Deaths From Other Causes	C Rehospitalized at Least Once for Heart Disease and Survived	D Living, Not Rehospitalized for Heart Disease	E Severe Recurrence* (A+C)
	Percent(N)	Percent(N)	Percent(N)	Percent(N)	Percent(N)
Under 40 (33)	21.2 (7)	3.0 (1)	27.3 (9)	48.5 (16)	48.5 (16)
40-44 (42)	26.2 (11)	2.4 (1)	19.0 (8)	52.4 (22)	45.2 (19)
45-49 (74)	17.6 (13)	5.4 (4)	20.3 (15)	56.8 (42)	37.9 (28)
50-54 (89)	18.0 (16)	2.2 (2)	24.7 (22)	55.1 (49)	42.7 (38)
55-60 (89)	29.2 (26)	3.4 (3)	16.8 (15)	50.6 (45)	46.0 (41)
Total (327)	22.3 (73)	3.4 (11)	21.1 (69)	53.2 (174)	43.4 (142)

*Severe recurrence is defined as rehospitalization and/or death due to heart disease. Men for whom we have incomplete information concerning rehospitalization are not included in the table. Period covered by table, it must be emphasized, is 8.0 years. Patients experiencing rehospitalization and/or death at a point such as 8.2 or 8.3 years are omitted from the computation. Hence, number of patients deceased differs from that recorded in Tables 2-1 and 2-3.

level, drawing upon measures from varying perspectives. These include physician assessments, subjective reports by patients on their health, and patient self-reports on their daily functioning and activities.

Physician Ratings at Year 8

Most of the men were described favorably by their physicians, in terms of their health level and their capacity for daily functioning. Of 140 men rated by their physicians, 66% were described as "able to engage in full activity without significant impairment."[2] Fourteen percent were classified as "able to engage in full activity but with significant modifications in his daily living schedule and activities." The 20% in the most serious condition were rated as having "definite residual limitations on his work and other activities."[3]

With regard to their present cardiac status, 46% of those patients rated by their physicians were described as being in the most favorable health category, i.e., "uncompromised." Thirty-three percent were rated "slightly compromised" and 18% "moderately compromised." The most serious condition, "severely compromised," described only five men, about 3% of the total.

On the whole, the physicians appeared to have a rather optimistic assessment of the status and prospects of the patients they rated. When asked to estimate "cardiac prognosis" on the basis of "an assessment of the potential effects of optimal current medical and surgical therapies," the physicians responded as follows: prognosis "good," 44% of the patients; "good with therapy," 29%; "fair with therapy," 15%; and "guarded despite therapy," 12%. Thus 73% of the patients were rated as being in the two most favorable prognostic categories.

Hospitalization History

One useful measure of health history is the incidence of hospitalization. It is an objective indicator of an event, and it is usually tied to medical judgment that a patient had a level of illness or a condition sufficiently serious to require such care. We can consider here the 205 surviving patients who were seen in four full interviews and from whom we have more detailed data than for others in the study.

Nearly one-fifth (19%) of the 205 patients had been hospitalized within the year prior to the Year 8 interview. Another 25% had been hospitalized in the period from 1 to 3 years prior to the last interview. At the other extreme, about 45% had not been in the hospital for 5 years or more; this number includes those who were never rehospitalized after the first heart attack. Of the total hospitalizations, about two-thirds were for heart disease.

A substantial proportion of the patients had experienced multiple rehospitalizations after Year 1. For the 205 men, the number of hospitalizations after Year 1 was as follows: one, 26%; two, 16%; three, 10%; four or more, 11%. These figures include both heart-related and non-heart-related admissions. Considering only rehospitalizations for heart disease, 18% of the surviving patients had one; 6% had two; 5% had three; and 6% had four or more. The latter group includes men with a particularly severe health history. Seven patients had been rehospitalized for heart disease six times or more since Year 1.

Symptoms During the Previous Month

Another perspective on health status of the patient population is furnished by reports from the patients themselves in regard to symptoms which they experienced during the previous month. Although patient perceptions obviously do not have the clarity and apparent precision of a laboratory test, it is useful to note that in classic diagnosis and treatment what the patient tells the doctor about his symptoms is an important criterion and point of reference in medical judgments. The significance and limitations of self-reported symptoms have been widely reviewed in numerous health behavior studies (Becker, 1979; Mechanic, 1978).

At Year 8 patients were asked questions about a list of 17 common symptoms, some of which are among the core items for diagnosis and treatment of heart disease (see Table 2–5). Since those who are most ill will presumably report the most frequent symptoms, we have divided the population into two levels of severity of heart disease as a control procedure: "recent heart

Table 2-5. Reported Symptoms Experienced at Least
Once in Month Preceding Year 8 Interview

| | *Percent Reporting Symptom** | | |
| | | | |
Reported Symptom	*Total Population* (N=205)	*Recent Heart Rehospitalization* (N=24)[†]	*No Recent Rehospitalization* (N=164)[†]
Getting Tired Easily	49.7 (102)	62.5 (15)	46.9 (77)
Chest Pain	29.7 (61)	37.5 (9)	29.9 (49)
Breathlessness	34.2 (70)	45.8 (11)	33.5 (55)
Feeling Heart Is Pounding	23.9 (49)	20.8 (5)	25.6 (42)
Swelling of Feet or Ankles	8.3 (17)	8.3 (2)	6.7 (11)
Sleeplessness	35.1 (72)	50.0 (12)	33.5 (55)
Restlessness or Nervousness	57.0 (117)	75.0 (18)	53.1 (87)
Upset Stomach	25.9 (53)	33.3 (8)	24.4 (40)
Headaches	28.3 (58)	25.0 (6)	28.1 (46)
General Aches and Pains	30.3 (62)	20.8 (5)	30.5 (50)
Loss of Appetite	8.3 (17)	16.7 (4)	7.3 (12)
Hands or Feet Shaking	10.2 (21)	8.3 (2)	9.7 (16)
Spells of Dizziness	17.5 (36)	20.8 (5)	18.3 (30)
Fainting Spells	1.5 (3)	4.2 (1)	1.2 (2)
Cold Sweats	13.7 (28)	12.5 (3)	13.4 (22)
Pains from Arthritis	20.0 (41)	12.5 (3)	19.5 (32)
Crying Spells	2.0 (4)	8.3 (2)	1.2 (2)
Other	22.0 (45)	25.0 (6)	20.1 (33)

*"Recent heart rehospitalization" includes all patients rehospitalized for
heart disease during the year preceding the Year 8 interview. "No recent
rehospitalization" includes all those not rehospitalized for any cause during that year. Percentages for the "recent heart rehospitalization" group
should be interpreted with particular caution because of the small base N.

[†]Columns 2 and 3 do not sum to 205, as men recently rehospitalized for
causes other than heart disease were excluded in this special analysis.

rehospitalization"—those who had been rehospitalized for heart disease within the preceding year; and "no recent rehospitalization"—those who had not been rehospitalized for heart disease or any other condition during the preceding year. Such a selection procedure allows for a more sensitive perspective on the self-reports by patients with somewhat differing recent patterns of heart disease: acute and not acute.[4]

As column 1 in Table 2–5 shows, the most prominent reported symptoms—"restlessness or nervousness"—suggest tension and anxiety. "Sleeplessness" also ranks high. "Getting tired easily" is also prominent. This symptom perhaps may seem innocuous for a population of older men, but it has more serious implications for a heart patient population. "Chest pains" and "breathlessness," classic symptoms of heart disease, also rank high.

Not surprisingly, those who were recently severely ill reported more symptoms than those men who were not recently hospitalized. However, several other features of Table 2–5 deserve note.

First, large proportions of men in both the "recent heart rehospitalization" and the "no recent rehospitalization" groups do not report key symptoms during the previous month. Thus, in this population of men with chronic cardiovascular disease, the *majority* report no chest pain the previous month, no breathlessness, and no feeling of disturbance of the rhythm of the heart. Of particular interest is the fact that this pattern is evident even among those who have been most recently hospitalized for heart disease.

At the same time, many symptoms were reported by considerable proportions of those not recently hospitalized. In most instances, in fact, the percentages of "recent heart rehospitalization" and "no recent rehospitalization" patients reporting a given symptom differs little.

Symptom Burden During the Previous Month

A simple additive index of number of symptoms reported can be useful as one means of describing the total "burden of symptoms" patients were experiencing at Year 8. Of course, mere numbers cannot truly approximate actual degrees of impairment or severity of illness. One significant symptom experienced daily may be far more indicative of serious impairment than four or five minor symptoms experienced three times a month. Nevertheless, a tabulation can serve to differentiate at least roughly those with the lightest symptom burden from those with the greatest.

We consider first those men whose symptoms were the most frequent, those who reported experiencing particular symptoms 3 days or more during the previous month.

Within the total cohort, the following percentages of men reported having symptoms 3 or more days during the month: Five symptoms or more on 3 or more days: 16.1% of the patients; three or four symptoms: 22%; one or two symptoms: 33.2%. The remaining 28.8% reported no symptoms which occurred on 3 or more days.

Aside from consideration of symptoms burden classified in terms of multiple occurrences during the previous month, we can gain another perspective on health level by considering the numbers of patients who had multiple symptoms. Thus, here we can tabulate the total number of patients who reported symptoms experienced at least once during the previous month. Such a tabulation revealed the following pattern: 6.8% of the patients reported no symptoms; 24.0% experienced one or two; 28.3% three or four; 23.0%, five or six; 18%, seven or more.

By their own reports, therefore, it would appear that for a considerable proportion of the study population life during the previous month involved experiencing multiple symptoms. And a considerable proportion had symptoms on 3 days or more of that month.

Age and Symptoms

In numerous studies, health level, as measured by reported symptoms, has been found to be associated with age. In our study population we found no relationship between age and number of reported symptoms. As we have noted earlier in another context, this lack of association may be related to the limited age range of the study population.

Examination of the full range of individual symptom items at Year 8 was handicapped by small numbers. However, for a series of items with appropriate distributions adequate for analysis, presence or absence of symptoms during the previous month was examined in relation to age level. These were "tiring easily," "chest pain," "breathlessness," "heart pounding," "restlessness, nervousness," and "sleeplessness." No statistically significant relationship with age was found. Thus, it is not useful simply to assume that the distribution of patients by age can serve somehow to account for the symptom patterns reported in this chapter.

Total Days of Pain or Discomfort

Another measure of health status is the number of days during a month when the patient experiences pain or discomfort. Like many other health measures, this indicator relies on highly subjective perceptions, and variable accuracy of reporting, as well as on the "objective" presence of pain and discomfort. Further, the mere occurrence of the symptoms does not necessarily indicate serious illness. Loss of appetite 3 days per month obviously has different implication than chest pain 3 days per month. Similarly, repeated headaches over the course of a month may have grave implications, but repeated sleeplessness alone is rarely life threatening. Even with these limitations, a simple differentiation by "symptom days" helps describe the health experience of this study population at a time long after the first heart attack.

The men were asked, "During the past month on how many days altogether did you experience any of the kinds of pains or discomforts that we just talked about?" Only a small proportion (6.8%) responded "None." Another 34% were also at the low end of the range, stating they felt pain or discomfort from 1 to 4 days of the previous month. Twelve percent reported such symptoms for from 5 to 7 days. At the upper end of the range, 26% stated they had pain or discomfort for 25 or more days of the month. The remaining population reported frequencies of pain or discomfort ranging from 8 through 24 days. While these data do not specify persistence, intensity, location, or seriousness of the pain or discomfort, it is apparent that for a large proportion of these men such feelings were a usual part of their lives. For over one-fourth of the men, symptoms were virtually a daily experience.

Performance of Everyday Activities

In performance of a series of specific, everyday activities—walking, climbing stairs, carrying weights, and driving—the patient population again presents a relatively favorable picture, having experienced only minimal impairment. Performance of the activities is clearly mediated by many factors. Those with the most severe cardiac residual limitations will obviously have the most difficulty. Aging, too, inevitably limits physical agility, and the effects of an habitually sedentary life may be reflected as well. Over two-fifths of the men (45%) reported no difficulty at all with any of the activities. The percentages reporting some difficulty were: lifting or carrying weights, 36%; climbing stairs or inclines, 36%; walking on level ground, 15.6%; driving, 7.0%. Of those citing difficulties, two-thirds mentioned only one; a few ($N = 18$) mentioned three or four.

It is perhaps most noteworthy that in the case of each activity in turn, most men reported no difficulty. For example, two-thirds of the men reported they had no problem in carrying weights in the course of their daily activities. The picture is similar with regard to climbing stairs. A small core of patients, 6%, noted they could not climb any stairs without symptoms, and an additional 14% reported that one flight of stairs was their limit. Seventeen percent indicated that they could climb no more than two flights without symptoms. These men together constitute nearly one-third of the total population. The remainder, however, indicated they could climb three flights or more without symptoms. In a population of elderly men with a history of heart disease, this finding must be viewed as relatively favorable.

Days of Illness and Impairment

It is notable that pain or malaise generally did not interfere significantly with the normal daily activities of the men at Year 8. This is evident in part from answers to the question, "On how many days during the past month were you unable to do your usual work at home or on the job because of pain or discomfort?"

Only a small minority reported being handicapped in their ordinary functioning by pain or discomfort. As many as 85%

stated there were *no* days when they could not carry out usual activities. Six percent reported being handicapped by pain or discomfort for from 1 to 3 days. These two groups alone account for over 90% of the population interviewed at Year 8. Less than 10% were impaired 4 days or more during the month.

These responses include impairment for any cause. If we look at restricted activity attributed to the heart condition in particular, the percentages are, of course, even smaller. Thus, only 15 (7%) of the 205 men reported that their heart condition limited their usual activities in the previous month. Two percent reported heart-related limitation on 1 to 3 days; 2% on 4 to 9 days; and 3% on 10 days or more.

We must emphasize that this measure is based on each patient's own frame of reference rather than on a standardized measure of impairment. A key factor here, of course, is that "usual work" is not defined, and we rely on the patient to make the appropriate definition in describing his life.

For many patients, therefore, "usual activity" may have been "scaled-down" activity, in order to adapt to their health condition. Consequently, the "usual activity" may actually be a degree of reduced functioning imposed by illness, age, or other factors. Within this context, however, a substantial majority of patients apparently believe they are able to perform fairly well.

Health Level and Bed Days

Finally, as a measure of health level, we can look at the number of days the patients reported spending in bed because of illness during the previous year. These data are presented in Table 2–6, classified by both cardiac and noncardiac causes. As can be seen, 40% of the study population did spend time in bed because of illness. However, most reported being ill in bed for 5 days or less.

Bed rest for heart-related illness alone was reported by only 14% of the total population. Of the 29 men so reporting, nearly half ($N = 12$) had bed rest for 5 days or less during the previous year. The next highest group ($N = 7$) were confined to bed 26 or more days because of heart disease.

To what extent is this pattern of reported symptoms, days of impairment, and bed days a function of age? At Year 8 do these

Table 2-6.   Disability As Measured by Reported Bed Days
in Year Preceding Year 8 Interview.
Total Population at Year 8.

Number of Bed Days	*Percent of Total Year 8 Population*		
	All Causes	Heart Disease[*]	Non-Cardiac Conditions[*]
None	59.5 (122)	85.8 (176)	70.2 (144)
1-5	23.9 (49)	5.9 (12)	19.5 (40)
6-10	5.4 (11)	1.5 (3)	4.4 (9)
11-15	3.4 (7)	2.4 (5)	1.0 (2)
16-20	1.4 (3)	.5 (1)	1.0 (2)
21-25	1.0 (2)	.5 (1)	1.0 (2)
26 or More	5.4 (11)	3.4 (7)	2.9 (6)
Total	100.0 (205)	100.0 (205)	100.0 (205)

[*]Some patients reported bed days for both heart and non-cardiac causes.

phenomena appear more marked among the older age groups than among the younger?

As we have seen, because of the rather favorable health experience of this population, the number of men with bed days or impairment days because of heart disease is small. The limited numbers inhibit meaningful statistical analysis. When categories are combined, however, no statistical association appears between age at Year 8 and number of bed days or impairment days because of heart disease. And as we have seen, no statistical association was found between (1) age at Year 8 and number of symptoms or (2) between age and number of days on which symptoms were experienced during the previous month.

HEALTH STATUS AT YEAR 8: AN EXPLORATION OF ANTECEDENTS AND "PREDICTORS"

In this longitudinal report on the heart patients, we have examined some key aspects of mortality, rehospitalization, and health status characteristics for a period extending over 8 years. We now turn to inquire whether there were clues in the backgrounds and histories of these patients which might have served as possible "predictors" of their current health status.

One way of approaching this question is to examine some variables which may be statistically associated with differing patterns of mortality, rehospitalization, and health status. We turn first to age, occupational level, educational status, selected psychological characteristics, and earlier indicators of health status. In other words, in this study population is age at the first myocardial infarction a significant variable in determining longterm health outcome? Do men from differing occupational backgrounds or educational levels have significantly different longterm health outcomes? Are psychological characteristics related to health over the long term? And how important a factor is the patient's health level early in the heart disease process in helping predict health status 8 years later?

Identifying the correlates of long-term health outcomes links also with questions concerning factors associated with the *etiology* of heart disease. At present, research and speculation abound in regard to the role of demographic, social, and psychological factors in the initial development of heart disease (Jenkins, 1971; Jenkins et al., 1974). Our research deals exclusively with men who have already developed heart disease, of course, and the issue of etiology itself is outside the scope of this study. However, questions raised by the problem of etiology can also be seen as relevant to the problems of (1) the recurrence of acute episodes and (2) the long-term course of the disease.

For example, if occupational level is associated with the development of the first heart attack, does it continue as a factor associated with the recurrence of the acute episodes? If men with particular psychological characteristics have high risk for developing the disease, is psychological status a continuing influence when the disease is well established, affecting later incidence of acute episodes? If, for example, as studies have suggested, a coronary-prone personality affects the development of the disease, are those heart patients with the most marked "coronaryprone" characteristics more likely than others to have a second heart attack and a poorer course of recovery (Alexander, 1950;

Jenkins, Zyzanski, & Rosenman, 1976)? Are such men in a population of heart patients particularly likely to suffer the more severe consequences of the heart disease? Thus, although we cannot cast any light on matters concerning etiology, our data do permit exploration of possible relationships between some hypothesized "etiological factors" and long-term mortality and morbidity measures.

Aside from the possible continuing role of social or psychological "etiological" factors, the issue of correlates of mortality and morbidity among heart patients raises another basic question. Various studies have reported apparent inverse relationships between coronary disease mortality and social status indicators. While the evidence is not conclusive, some data suggest that survival records may be especially poor among men with low education, low income, and with few occupational skills (Comstock, 1971; Hrubec & Zukel, 1971; Shapiro et al., 1970; Weinblatt et al., 1978).

Such evidence on heart disease mortality is consistent, of course, with general epidemiological findings on differences in mortality and morbidity rates among people from differing positions in the social structure (Antonovsky, 1967; Kitagawa & Hauser, 1973). While the exact connection between social status and heart disease is unclear, there are numerous leads and hypotheses, based on informed speculation (Buell & Eliot, 1979; Jenkins, 1978b). In the context of this developing body of information and research, we report on the long-term fate of the total study population, considering the possible association of social status factors.

Our first report (Croog & Levine, 1977), reviewed data on the medical fate of patients covering the first year following the heart attack. We now turn to the period subsequent to Year 1, extending approximately 7 years to Year 8. We also take a comprehensive approach to the two phases of this study, combining the data for the full 8-year study period. Our examination of long-term health outcomes uses several measures:

(1)   mortality from heart disease or survival during the period from Year 1 to Year 8

(2) the prevalence of "severe recurrence" during the period from Year 1 to Year 8[5]

(3) physicians' ratings of "cardiac status" of the patients at Year 8[6]

(4) self-reported symptoms experienced during the month preceding the Year 8 interview[7]

Each of these measures provides data from somewhat differing perspectives on health as of Year 8: (1) the objective facts of death or survival and rehospitalization, (2) physicians' assessments, and (3) the patients' perceptions. (Another measure of health outcome, "functional health status" as rated by physicians, is examined in Chapter 8 in the context of review of variables on behavior and performance "outcomes.")

Age and Health Outcome

For purposes of this analysis, age of patients at entry into the study was classified into five categories: under 40, 40 to 44, 45 to 49, 50 to 54, and 55 to 60. In some instances, special analysis employing age as a control reduced the numbers in cells and made it necessary to combine categories. In such cases, the population was divided into two groups: (1) 49 and under, and (2) 50 and over.

The question of the relationship between age and "health outcome" has already been touched upon earlier in this chapter. As we noted, no statistical association was found between age and mortality and acute recurrences for the 8-year period following entry into the study.[8]

Findings are mixed in regard to other outcome measures. No statistical association appeared between age and the physician's assessment of the cardiac status of patients at Year 8. Age was related to some self-reported problems, such as difficulty in climbing stairs. However, neither total number of symptoms reported nor pattern of symptoms varied by age. In sum, in this study population the age variable did not appear to be a major differentiating factor in accounting for health outcome with the measures employed here.

Health Outcomes and Social Status Measures: Education, Occupation, and Income Level

The Base-Line Study.   In our earlier study covering the year following the first heart attack (1977), we reported that "physical health outcomes" were not significantly related to such measures of social status as educational level, occupational level, and income. However, we noted some indications of possible associations which could deserve further inquiry in a long-term, follow-up study.

At the close of that first year the number of heart-related deaths was relatively small ($N = 14$). It was thus not possible to carry out detailed analysis of mortality and social status measures. For exploratory purposes we therefore combined (1) deaths from heart disease and (2) the number of surviving men who suffered one or more additional heart attacks during the year. We designated this population as consisting of men with "severe recurrences," i.e., persons with one or more acute cardiac episodes resulting in rehospitalization and/or death.

Considering men classified by three measures of socioeconomic status (occupational level, education, and income) some consistent themes emerged in regard to "severe recurrences" in the first year. Men at the top level of all three scales did somewhat better than others, remaining the most "healthy" throughout the year. Men at the bottom of the three scales did somewhat worse. On all three measures there was consistent ranking by occupation, education, and income levels in regard to the prevalence of severe recurrences. Thus, although there were no statistically significant differences, the data implied that the cardiac health status of the men during the year might be related to position in the social structure. In terms of health alone, it seemed preferable to be a highly educated, high-income professional or executive, rather than a low-income, semiskilled, or unskilled worker with 3 years or less of high school education.

The Follow-Up Study.   Completion of the full follow-up study presents a fortunate opportunity to pursue our inquiry into the questions raised by the data from Year 1. We focus first on the relationship between mortality from heart disease and indicators of social status of 8 years. The results are shown in Table 2–7.

The table offers suggestive themes similar to findings of the earlier study. Although data on occupational level and deaths from coronary disease show no linear relationship, the extremes of the occupational categories deserve note. The professionals and high level executives had the most favorable survival rate for the 8 years, and the percentage who died of heart disease in particular is lowest in this occupational group (14.3%). In contrast, nearly one-third of the semiskilled and unskilled workers died of heart disease, and the proportion of total survivors was lowest. A chi-square comparison of the semiskilled and unskilled workers with other occupational categories revealed that they differed significantly. In turn, a comparison of the executives and professionals with all other occupational categories resulted in a chi-square in the direction of significance. (p < .10).

Data on the patients when arrayed by income level at the start of the study show a somewhat similar pattern in terms of a suggestive underlying trend. The proportion of deaths due to heart disease shows a weak increment as one moves down the income scale, but there is no significant difference between the coronary deceased and the survivors. Heart-related deaths range from 16.2% for the highest income group to 30% for the lowest. When the lowest income group was compared with all others on the chi-square test, a finding consistent with the occupational level finding appeared: the lowest income men differed significantly from all others in terms of cardiac mortality (p < .05). However, the highest income group did not significantly differ from the remaining population.

In contrast to the data on occupation and income, the materials on educational level revealed no trend toward association with cardiac mortality. This finding is somewhat surprising, given the common association between occupational level, income, and education. (See Table 2–7 a,b,c.)

We next examined the 8-year data in regard to the social status variables and the incidence of at least one severe recurrence. The procedure was consistent with the one followed for our study of the base-line year. However, the suggestive trends in the earlier study did not emerge. No relationships were found be-

Table 2-7a. Social Status and Mortality During Eight Years After First Heart
Attack: Occupational Level

Occupational Level*	(1) Deaths Due to Heart Disease Percent (N)	(2) Deaths Due to Other Causes Percent (N)	(3) Survivors Percent (N)	Total Study Group (Number of Patients)
A. High Level Executives or Professionals	14.3 (9)	3.2 (2)	82.5 (52)	63
B. Upper White Collar	23.9 (11)	4.4 (2)	71.7 (33)	46
C. Lower White Collar	20.8 (15)	5.6 (4)	73.6 (53)	72
D. Skilled Blue Collar	21.0 (13)	1.6 (1)	77.4 (48)	62
E. Semiskilled and Unskilled Blue Collar	31.6 (31)	3.1 (3)	65.3 (64)	98
Total	79	12	250	341†

*See Note 1 in Chapter 3 for definitions of occupational categories.
†Patients were omitted from analysis if information concerning survival status, cause of death or occupational level was incomplete.

Column 1 versus Columns 2 and 3: Heart-Deceased vs. Medical Fate Other Than Heart-Deceased
A,B,C,D,E (Total Group) Chi-square = 7.14, d.f. = 4, p<.20
A vs. B,C,D,E (Highest vs. All Other) Chi-square = 2.84, d.f. = 1, p<.10
E vs. A,B,C,D (Lowest vs. All Other) Chi-square = 4.89, d.f. = 1, p<.05

Table 2-7b. Social Status and Mortality During Eight Years After First Heart Attack: Educational Level

Educational Level	(1) Deaths Due to Heart Disease Percent (N)	(2) Deaths Due to Other Causes Percent (N)	(3) Survivors Percent (N)	Total Study Group (Number of Patients)
A. One Year of College or More	18.1 (15)	3.6 (3)	78.3 (65)	83
B. High School Graduate	26.6 (29)	5.5 (6)	67.9 (74)	109
C. Completed Grades 10-11	22.7 (15)	1.5 (1)	75.8 (50)	66
D. Completed Grade 9 or Less	24.4 (20)	2.4 (2)	73.2 (60)	82
Total	79	12	249	340*

*Patients were omitted from analysis if information concerning survival status, cause of death, or educational level was incomplete.

Column 1 versus Columns 2 and 3: Heart-Deceased vs. Medical Fate Other Than Heart-Deceased
A vs. B,C,D (Most Education vs. All Others)   Chi-square = 1.28, d.f. = 1, NS
D vs. A,B,C (Least Education vs. All Others)   Chi-square = .02, d.f. = 1, NS

60

Table 2-7c. Social Status and Mortality During Eight Years After First Heart Attack: Total Family Income

	(1) Deaths Due to Heart Disease Percent (N)	(2) Deaths Due to Other Causes Percent (N)	(3) Survivors Percent (N)	Total Study Group (Number of Patients)
Total Family Income				
A. $15,000 or More	16.2 (6)	5.4 (2)	78.4 (29)	37
B. $12,500–14,999	17.2 (5)	(0)	82.8 (24)	29
C. $10,000–12,499	19.6 (11)	1.8 (1)	78.6 (44)	56
D. $7,500–9999	21.5 (23)	4.7 (5)	73.8 (79)	107
E. Less Than $7500	30.0 (33)	3.6 (4)	66.4 (73)	110
Total	78	12	249	339*

*Patients were omitted from analysis if information concerning survival status, cause of death, or total family income was incomplete.

Column 1 versus Columns 2 and 3: Heart-Deceased vs. Medical Fate Other Than Heart-Deceased
A,B,C,D,E (Total Group)   Chi-square = 5.04, d.f. = 4, p<.30, NS
E vs. A,B,C,D (Lowest Income vs. All Others)   Chi-square = 3.93, d.f. = 1, p<.05
A vs. B,C,D,E (Highest Income vs. All Others)   Chi-square = .69, d.f. = 1, NS

tween total severe recurrences and occupation, education, or income level. In other words, only those data on the clear-cut phenomenon of death or survival appeared to have possible meaning when social status variables were considered.

Might these suggestive differences on heart disease mortality be explained simply by age differences between the various occupational and income level subgroups? Our investigation showed no significant age differences between the subgroups. In any case, as we saw earlier, no association was found between age and coronary death in this study population.

In sum, as we have noted, our own previous study, national and historical data on mortality rates, and other research on heart patients suggested we might find possible associations between long-term mortality and social status characteristics. Some emergent indications indeed appeared when we examined mortality in relation to occupational level and income level. The findings on the problems of the lower occupational and income groups seem strongest; they are also consistent with other findings in this report in regard to the special difficulties faced by low-income, blue-collar patients. At the other extreme of the occupational scale, executives and professionals appeared to have the most favorable health careers over the 8 years of this study.

But these findings emerged only in regard to the heart disease mortality and survival data. They did not appear when our measure of morbidity—"severe recurrence"—was employed. This may have been due to the possibility that "severe recurrence" is simply too inclusive a term for use in classifying complex phenomena involving multiple infarctions, impairment, and disability. Further, though others have found educational level to be a useful differentiating variable in research analogous to ours, its lack of association with cardiac mortality-survival is noteworthy in this study.

Self-Rated Psychological Characteristics and Long-Term Health Outcomes

As psychological characteristics have received increasing attention as possible factors in the etiology of heart disease, it seems also relevant to ask whether they are related to long-term health outcomes among persons who have become heart patients. We approach this question through use of a series of psychological self-rating items employed earlier in the base-line study.

Patients were asked during the interview to characterize themselves in regard to each of a series of items.[9] These included a number of variables often characterized as related to a coronary-prone behavior pattern, such as "being in a hurry," "ambition," "eating rapidly," "liking responsibility," and others involving competitivness, aggression and time-urgency (Friedman & Rosenman, 1974; Haynes et al., 1978a & b; Jenkins, 1971).* At Week 7 we asked the men to rate themselves as they had been before the heart attack, some weeks earlier. At Year 1 they rated themselves in terms of their current characteristics.

In the base-line study, individual ratings by patients concerning the pre-illness period and Year 1 were highly similar (Croog & Levine, 1977). Further, we found that patients' self-ratings and the ratings of the men by their wives were highly associated both for the pre-illness period and for Year 1 (Croog, Koslowsky, & Levine, 1976). There thus appeared to be some marked consistency in the manifestation of these characteristics over time.

In addition to analyzing individual self-rating items, we carried out a factor analysis of the items for the pre-illness period and for Year 1 in order to help develop a descriptive picture of the underlying dimensions. These results have been reported in detail elsewhere (Croog & Levine, 1977; Croog, Koslowsky & Levine, 1976). The three most prominent factors in the base-line study can be identified as "emotional lability," "dominance," and "ambition."

For purposes of the present study, we examined psychological self-rating responses for both pre-illness and Year 1 in relation to the health outcome variables at Year 8. In addition, to achieve greater economy in analysis, we also examined the pre-illness factor scores rated at Week 7 in relation to the health outcome variables at Year 8.

*It should be stressed that our methodology differs from that employed by other investigators and that our items cannot be interpreted as measures of Type A in the sense of the construct as measured by Rosenman and Friedman interviews or by the Jenkins scale.

The results can be summarized briefly in general terms. On the whole, individual psychological characteristics for both pre-illness and Year 1 were not significantly associated with health outcome measures at Year 8, such as (1) mortality, (2) rehospitalization for heart disease, (3) the combined measure, "severe recurrences," or (4) physicians' ratings of cardiac status of the patients at Year 8. Examination of the psychological factor scores in relation to health outcome measures produced essentially the same lack of association.

Sole exceptions were found in regard to relationships between a number of pre-illness psychological items and symptoms at Year 8. For example, patients who had earlier rated themselves as "nervous or irritable" reported more symptoms at Year 8: 78% of patients who rated themselves as "high" on this psychological variable reported the presence of three or more symptoms 8 years later as compared with 50% of those who had described themselves as "not at all nervous or irritable." Those who said they were "easily depressed" at Week 7 were most likely to report "sleeplessness" at Year 8. Thus, it appears that men who had problems of mood according to one set of measures had similar kinds of symptoms 8 years later. Aside from this finding, no relationships were seen between psychological characteristics and individual physical symptoms, such as chest pain or shortness of breath.

In this discussion of psychological status and health outcomes, we wish to emphasize that, in the main, our report makes use of individual items rather than scales. Work by others in this field (Haynes, et al., 1978a & b; Jenkins et al., 1974) has generally employed scales. The product of data from individual items and from scale scores cannot be systematically compared. This might explain some of the puzzling differences between our findings and those of others with regard to the possibility of long-term association between psychological factors and health outcomes in heart disease. However, the whole issue deserves further study.

The Issue of Work Stress: Heart Disease Deaths and Rehospitalizations

"Hard work never killed anybody!" So states the ancient aphorism. Whatever the general applicability of the folk saying may be, its underlying thesis has long been suspect as far as heart disease is concerned. Although the role of work in the etiology of heart disease is not clear, numerous elements have been identified as possibly implicated (Antonovsky, 1967; House, 1975; Jenkins, 1976). These include objective physical factors which produce excessive sudden and/or continuous stresses on heart muscle and the cardiovascular system, such as heavy lifting, noxious environmental conditions, and chemical hazards. They include also various types of psychosocial stresses, including heavy work load, long working hours, role conflict, multiple responsibilities, interpersonal stresses, status incongruity, and lack of gratification and rewards on the job.

Physical stresses at work have long been regarded by the medical and legal systems as of etiological importance in the development of heart disease (Wenger & Hellerstein, 1978). We have even seen the development of "heart laws" in recent years which assume that in the case of particular occupational groups— such as police and firemen—heart disease is a consequence of the hazards of their work, and they are accordingly entitled to appropriate disability ratings on that basis. However, the role of psychosocial stresses in heart disease has been subject to particular controversy. Although a substantial body of laboratory and field research evidence now exists, the underlying factors still have not been delineated, and conflicting findings and hypotheses still remain to be resolved on a scientific basis.

After patients have had at least one myocardial infarction, does work stress constitute a risk factor for further recurrences of the acute phase? In other words, are heart patients with a history of high work stress at particular risk for subsequent death and/or rehospitalization from heart disease? These questions follow from the hypotheses which hold that work stresses are related to etiology in the first place, although they are not necessarily dependent on the validity of these hypotheses. Given our findings on the higher rate of death from heart disease among the semi- and unskilled men over the course of 8 years, we thought it appropriate to explore the possibility that such findings might be related to stress conditions of their work.

We examined the relation of work stress to cardiac mortality and morbidity in several ways. We first asked whether evidence of work stress before the first heart attack constituted a risk factor for long-term survival and/or rehospitalization. Several measures of pre-illness work stress were used. These were: (1) the number of hours worked per week by the patient before the first heart attack; (2) score on a work stress index, comprised of items drawn from the Midtown Manhattan study; (3) a patient's belief that work stress contributed to his heart attack, including both physical stresses at work and emotional tensions; and (4) report of physical activity at work, such as frequency of heavy lifting. Thus, these measures comprise a series of indicators from differing perspectives—from the standpoint of physical and emotional work load, subjective work stresses, and perceptions that particular types of stresses were severe enough to cause a heart attack.

In a second approach, we centered on the patient at Year 1. Here we used essentially the same measures as listed above, except that information was collected in regard to current work stresses and beliefs at Year 1. The variable on numbers of hours worked is not part of the analysis of the Year 1 data, as information was not collected on the topic at the time.

In the analysis here we employed the items both singly and in combinations. Details on the individual items appear in Chapter 3, where we discuss issues pertaining to work experience over the years.

The results can be simply summed up: no relationships were found between our pre-illness and Year 1 work stress measures and mortality and morbidity over the 8 years of the study. Further, the data on work stresses did not explain the high mortality among the semiskilled and unskilled workers, as compared with other occupational groups. We carried out special analyses controlling for level of work stress pre-illness and at Year 1, comparing the fate of the semiskilled and unskilled workers with men in other occupational levels and no differences were found. Hence, these data suggest that we must look beyond any simple hypothesis that the semi-and unskilled workers died in higher proportions because they had greater physical and/or emotional stress on the job.

These negative results have some other aspects which deserve note. In general, the men in executive and professional occupations reported higher stress levels both for the pre-illness period and at Year 1. Yet this group, as we saw earlier, did not differ in mortality rate from the men in other occupational levels (Table 2–7a). In fact, the data suggested that their mortality rate was slightly lower than that of the others, although the differences were not statistically significant.

The materials here deal solely with the issue of work stress at two time points as a risk factor for subsequent deaths and/or rehospitalizations. They describe a select group of men with clinical cardiovascular disease who had already experienced the acute phase of the illness. We do not have data on fluctuations in the stresses over time or on idiosyncratic stressful events. Detailed analysis of ongoing stresses in the intervening periods between the time points might have produced other results more consistent with traditional hypotheses concerning stress and heart disease.

Illness Status During the First Year

Of the variables we examined, those most consistently related to long-term outcomes at Year 8 were indicators of severity of illness level during the year following the first myocardial infarction. In an actuarial sense, these indicators serve as possible "predictors" of later outcome, since those who reported more severe early illness had a higher probability of later negative health experience. In another sense, however, these data may be only describing the continuity of pathological process in the cardiovascular system. Thus, those men experiencing the most initially severe cardiac conditions continue to manifest them; their mortality, rehospitalization, and symptom record is accordingly less favorable than for those with less serious initial cardiac status.

At the same time, it must be emphasized that a considerable proportion of those who were at first most seriously ill did quite well over the long term. By the same token, some of those who were most mildly stricken subsequently suffered recurrence or even death over the years of the study. Thus, while the data suggest continuities in the pathological process of the disease, they also underline the unpredictable nature of the illness.

In our base-line study covering the first year, we found physicians' assessments of the patients' functional health status to be a most useful variable in analysis. The patients with the least favorable physicians' ratings, i.e., greatest impairment, had the highest rate of rehospitalization and death during the first year. With regard to the 7-year period from Year 1 to Year 8 as well, the physician assessment at Year 1 was a good predictor of subsequent health outcome. As Table 2–8 shows, among those rated as having no significant impairment at Year 1, approximately one-fifth were dead of heart disease at Year 8. Of those with the greatest impairment, however, 44% had died in the same period. The data on rehospitalization, as well as the combined data on severe recurrence (column D), reveal a similar picture.

Other indicators show the same basic pattern. Of those men rehospitalized for heart disease at least once during the first year, 66% had a severe recurrence during the period from Year 1 to Year 8; among those who were not rehospitalized, 43% had a severe recurrence (see Table 2–8). It is noteworthy, however, that the proportion of deaths from heart disease was approximately the same for men who were rehospitalized during the first year and for those who were not rehospitalized. Thus, difference in the percentage with "severe recurrence" (column D) is explained by difference in the rate of "rehospitalization with survival."

Another measure of health at Year 1 was the report by patients on whether they were depressed or discouraged because of the illness. As the table shows, patients who reported early depressive reaction about their illness also had less favorable medical fates at Year 8. The meaning of this finding is not clear. It may be influenced in part by personality factors, threshold for depression, and denial, as well as the objective seriousness of the illness. Indeed, it might be possible to explain the negative health outcome mainly on the grounds that the depressive reaction is part of the total syndrome of serious coronary illness. Thus, the most seriously ill heart patients at Year 1 are most likely (1) to be among the most seriously ill at Year 8 and (2) to be among those with the most intensive depressive reaction. However, it is also worth noting that other investigators have suggested that depression itself may be involved in the etiology of heart disease (Dreyfuss, Dasberg, & Assael, 1969; Eastwood & Trevelyan, 1971; Jenkins, 1978a; Thiel, Parker, & Bruce, 1973).

Finally, physicians' reports on cardiac status at Year 8 are consistent with the patterns reviewed above. The various mea-

Table 2-8. Severe Recurrence of Heart Disease Between Year 1 and Year 8 Interviews: By Illness Level at Year 1

Measure of Year 1 Illness Level	N*	Health Outcome as of Year 8			
		_A_ Deceased Due to Heart Disease Percent (N)	_B_ Rehospitalized at Least Once for Heart Disease and Survived Percent (N)	_C_ Other: No Severe Recurrence: No Death or Rehospitalization for Heart Disease# Percent (N)	_D_ Severe Recurrence (A+B) Percent (N)
Physician Rating of Functional Health Status					
Severe Impairment	32	43.8 (14)	34.4 (11)	21.8 (7)	78.2 (25)
Moderate Impairment	64	12.5 (8)	32.8 (21)	54.7 (35)	45.3 (29)
No Significant Impairment	146	19.8 (29)	21.2 (31)	59.0 (86)	41.0 (60)
			Chi-square = 20.28, d.f. = 4, p<.001		
Rehospitalization for Heart Disease During First Year					
Yes	44	22.7 (10)	43.2 (19)	34.1 (15)	65.9 (29)
No	240	20.8 (50)	22.5 (54)	56.7 (136)	43.3 (104)
			Chi-square = 9.81, d.f. = 2, p<.05		
Reported Depressive Reaction at Year 1†					
Yes	140	27.1 (38)	29.3 (41)	43.6 (61)	56.4 (79)
No	142	15.5 (22)	22.6 (32)	61.9 (88)	38.1 (54)
			Chi-square = 10.25, d.f. = 2, p<.01		

*Numbers vary due to incomplete data. See Note 2 on the pattern of completion of physician questionnaires.

†See also Chapter 7 for discussion of depressive reaction.

#"Other" includes men with miscellaneous health fates other than heart-related rehospitalization and/or death: (a) those who experienced rehospitalization and/or death for non-cardiac causes and (b) survivors without rehospitalization.

sures of earlier severity of the illness (physician rating at Year 1, rehospitalization during the first year, depressive reaction) are associated with cardiac status at Year 8. Reports of symptoms at Year 8 are similarly related to the earlier measures. For example, men classified by their physicians as "severely impaired" at Year 1 report more symptoms than the "least impaired" group during the month prior to the Year 8 interview.

What can we conclude from these materials on long-term health outcomes and the antecedent variables? Except for the limited findings on income and occupational differences in cardiac mortality, the data suggest that the underlying process of the illness continued to make itself evident over the 8 years. Thus, on the whole, demographic, social, and psychological items seemed less useful for explaining *physical* health outcomes than did the intrinsic nature of the illness and its physiological course.[10]

Demographic, social, and psychological types of variables do, however, play a very significant role in explaining the long-term *social and psychological sequelae* of the disease, differing *patterns of recovery*, and *barriers to rehabilitation*. The remaining chapters of this report will address these issues.

Multiple Regression Analysis and Long-Term Health Outcomes: An Addendum

In line with our general policy on data analysis for this study, the principal methods employed in this chapter rely on nonparametric statistics. In reviewing these data, however, the possibility remained that some underlying themes might be present which only more powerful statistical methods might bring forth. Hence, for exploratory purposes, we chose to carry out a multiple regression analysis, making use of the same independent and dependent variables employed in the nonparametric procedures.

This multiple regression analysis followed the conceptual format of this chapter in many respects, assessing the relative importance of medical, social, and demographic variables in long-term health outcomes. The results were consistent with the findings using nonparametric statistics. (See Appendix B for further details.)

SUMMARY

In examining the morbidity and mortality experience of the heart patient study population, we reviewed data for a total study period extending over 8 years. In the year following their first heart attack, almost over one-fourth of the men had either died or had been rehospitalized for heart disease. By Year 8, half of the original population had suffered a cardiac "severe recurrence"—rehospitalization for heart disease and/or death. Since the first heart attack, three out of every four men in the original population had either died or had been rehospitalized at least once. Heart disease accounted for two-thirds of these cases.

The rate of death in the study group did not manifest a linear trend over the 8-year period examined. There was no significant relationship between age and risk of cardiac "severe recurrence" in this study population.

The health status of survivors at the Year 8 interview was generally favorable. Although many patients had been rehospitalized or suffered serious symptoms over the intervening years, we found minimal overall day-to-day disability. The great majority of the surviving patients experienced no limitations on their everyday activities, and relatively few experienced persistent symptoms related to their heart disease. Most had optimistic cardiac prognoses from their physicians.

When social status measures were examined in relation to the health outcomes at Year 8, mixed findings emerged. Over the full 8-year period, men with the lowest total family incomes and least skilled occupations had higher mortality due to heart disease than the rest of the study population. These findings are consistent with data from our base-line study which suggested that the cardiac health status of the patients in the first year might be related to their position in the social structure. However, there were no differences in cardiac mortality among men of differing educational levels.

No significant associations emerged between health status outcomes at Year 8 and age or self-rated psychological characteristics. Work stress before the first heart attack and at Year 1 was not found to be a significant risk factor for cardiac "severe recurrence" over the period to Year 8.

On the whole, social and psychological factors appeared less useful as predictors of long-term health outcomes at Year 8 than the severity of the disease as evidenced during the base-line study.

NOTES

1. Two types of "accounting" procedures are carried out in this chapter. The *first* reviews the characteristics of the patients over the course of the full study period in regard to the morbidity and mortality. The *second* involves a more limited focus on the mortality-morbidity data in the context of a specific time period, i.e., within 8.0 years since the first heart attack.

    The use of the two methods links back to our schedule of interviewing for the follow-up study, as explained in Chapter 1. In the base-line study we returned to interview each patient at 1 year after his first heart attack. Since the total period of case intake extended about 18 months, this meant that the Year 1 interview program necessarily had to last that long in order that patients would be seen on their 1-year anniversary date.

    For the current report at Year 8, it was not feasible to carry out an interview schedule which would extend the full 18 months. Limited funds, personnel, and time made it essential that the follow-up interview program be completed in about 1 year.

    As a consequence, some patients were interviewed on or about their anniversaries, while others were seen some months after their anniversaries. The distribution of interview or questionnaire contacts at Year 8 was as follows: 8.0 to 8.9 years after the first interview: 69.5%; 9.0 to 9.5 years: 30.5%. The mean interval from the first interview to the last was 8.7 years.

    This exigency limits the period for which we can say there was uniform surveillance. As of 8.0 years after the first interview, we had information about virtually all patients in regard to whether they were alive or dead, and in regard to previous hospitalization. However, we cannot state with certainty what proportion of patients were alive as of 9.0 years following the first interview. Hence, we choose 8.0 years as the delimited time period for our report on mortality.

    Given this contingency, we have made appropriate indications in the text of this chapter where the issue is relevant. We have also reported on patients for the total interview program from Week 3 to Year 8, although there is some variation in the length of the period. Our larger purpose here, as we have noted, is the review of the long-term recovery and rehabilitation experience of the heart patients. Our working assumption is that the social and psychological phenomena described in this report in the main will not be significantly affected by whether the patient is 8.7 years postentry into the study or 8.2 years postentry.

As a final note, we might point out that the two methods of accounting do not lead to significantly differing results.

2. The report on physician assessments is based upon a mail questionnaire. Of 205 patients in the interview program at Year 8, 148 full questionnaires were completed by the physicians (72%). The reasons for nonresponse are varied. Deliberate noncompliance by the physicans despite repeated follow-up letters and personal contacts accounted for only 13% ($N = 27$). In 7% of the cases ($N = 14$), no questionnaire was sent as the patient reported that he had no regular physician, or he had not seen the doctor in so long a time that no accurate address could be found. In seven cases the physician chose not to complete the questionnaire, explaining that he had not seen the patient recently and therefore could not respond. In two cases the physician had retired, and had no access to information on the patient. In three cases instructions for completion were not followed, and the materials could not be coded. In two cases the patient refused permission for his physician to be contacted.

3. Throughout this volume, for the sake of brevity, we will employ the following terms to designate ratings of functional health status by the physician: no significant impairment, moderate impairment, and severe impairment.

4. In order to minimize the confounding effects of hospitalization for other illnesses during the previous year, a number of patients who were hospitalized for noncardiac conditions have been omitted from this analysis.

5. As we have noted, "severe recurrence" is defined here as one or more acute cardiac episodes resulting in rehospitalizaton and/or death.

6. Following criteria of the New York Heart Association, the categor-

ies were "uncompromised," "slightly compromised" "moderately compromised," and "severely compromised" (New York Heart Association, 1973).

7. We examine both individual symptoms and an index of the total number of symptoms reported. The index was developed by division of the Year 8 population into three symptom groups: high, medium, and low.

8. In reporting of data on "health outcome" in the remaining sections of this chapter, we will refer to the period from Year 1 to Year 8, covering the period from the third interview to the time the fourth one was scheduled, unless otherwise specified. Data on outcomes from Week 3 to Year 1 have already been reported in our first book, *The Heart Patient Recovers* (1977). Further, in order to maximize numbers, we are reporting on the period to the Year 8 interview, rather than the period to 8.0 years. Findings for both periods are identical, in terms of statistical significance, unless otherwise specified. See also Note 1.

9. A more detailed description of the psychological self-rating methodology appears in Chapter 7. The psychological self-rating items were as follows: sense of humor, sense of duty, stubborn, gets angry easily, feelings easily hurt, nervous or irritable, easygoing, moody, jealous, likes to take responsibility, dominating or bossy, critical of others, easily excited, shy, likes belonging to organizatins, easily depressed, self-centered, in a hurry, ambitious, eats rapidly, hard driving, and puts a lot of effort into things.

10. For a listing of independent variables used in the analysis of morbidity and mortality at Year 8, and the dependent variables assessing disability and symptoms of illness, see Appendix C.

Chapter 3

WORK, FINANCES, AND THE COSTS
OF ILLNESS

WORK

Work is one of the key elements in the "armory of resources" for the heart patients in our study. It is highly valued in American society. Indeed, for American males, and increasingly for females, success in one's job tends to be of paramount importance in determining one's sense of worth. In our present study, as well as in our past base-line research, work has major significance in the lives of heart patients. While still recovering from their first heart attack in the hospital, a high proportion of patients devoted considerable attention to planning their return to work. Relatively soon after discharge, a marked proportion had returned or were planning to return to work (Croog & Levine, 1977).

Focus on the issue of "return to work" has been one of the most central themes in recent years in the literature on rehabilitation and recovery of heart patients. In these studies, many researchers have reported differing rates of return to work, and their data has been affected in part by the occupational classification of the patients, their severity of illness, the study design, and other factors. But, on the whole, the data show that high proportions of patients with first myocardial infarction return to their employment within 6 months (Doehrman, 1977; Garrity, 1973; Hammermeister et al., 1979; Shapiro, Weinblatt, & Frank, 1972).

Few data are available, however, on the long-term work careers of heart patients and on issues beyond the initial questions of work return and its correlates (Doehrman, 1977; Sanne, 1979). Using these data from our follow-up study after 8 years, we can document and describe some features of the work experience, job satisfaction, work stress and retirement in our study population.

This chapter presents findings of the follow-up study at Year 8, and compares them with our earlier findings concerning the pre-illness experience and Year 1. It must be emphasized that we are now considering those patients who are survivors at Year 8. As we observed in the previous chapter, an appreciable proportion of patients died over the course of the study. As we shall see, most surviving patients have continued working without too many negative consequences. A majority who kept working returned to their original places of work and adjusted fairly well. For the most part, their health seems not to have posed very serious obstacles to their ability to carry out their occupational roles, adjust to the requirements of the job, or maintain satisfactory relationships with employers and fellow employees. An appreciable minority of patients, however, report that poor health has had a negative effect on their work status or success on the job.

Employment Status at Year 8

Eight years after their first heart attacks, almost two-thirds of subjects participating in the final follow-up were working full time ($N = 130$). (See Table 3–1.) When we include those who are working part time, as well, we find that as many as 69% of participating survivors are gainfully employed at Year 8. For a majority of surviving patients, therefore, their heart conditions did not pose a serious barrier to employment.

This welcome finding, however, must be balanced against the fact that as many as one-fourth ($N = 51$) of our surviving subjects are retired, and an additional 6% ($N = 13$) are unemployed (see Table 3–1). Almost all retirements occurred between Year 1 and Year 8. Most noteworthy from our perspective is that 59% of those who retired did so primarily for reasons of ill health,

Table 3-1. Employment Status at Year 8

Employment Status	Number of Patients	Percent of Year 8 Study Population
Employed Full Time	130	63.4
Employed Part Time	11	5.4
Retired	51	24.9
Unemployed	13	6.3
Total	205	100.0

and an additional 9% for a combination of reasons including ill health. Only about 11% left the labor force solely because they had reached the age of retirement. Of those few categorized as unemployed, almost half (6 of 13) cited health as the reason for their unemployment. Thus, a quarter of the patients at Year 8 dropped out of work for health reasons.

One qualification is in order. The category of *retired* is not completely pure: retirement does not necessarily imply total withdrawal from the work force. Some of the men in our study retired and subsequently took other jobs. One quarter of the "retired" men answered that they still worked occasionally. Furthermore, those patients currently listed as unemployed will not necessarily continue to be unemployed. Eleven of the thirteen men unemployed at Year 8 indicated that they planned to return to work.

The majority of the participating heart patients at Year 8 ($N = 192$) indicated that they had worked at least part of the period between Year 1 and Year 8; only 6% had been unemployed the entire time. Though most (58%) of those who had worked since Year 1 had had only one employer, 34 men (16.6%) had had two employers and 16 men (7.9%) had had three to five employers. Three-quarters of the men (75.6%) reported working "full time only" since Year 1. Those who listed less than full-time employment frequently cited health reasons. Of the 30 men who reported some full-time and some part-time employment since Year 1, 20 attributed their limited employment to health. Of the seven who worked only part time, four gave health reasons.

Patients were also asked a series of questions about employment during the year immediately preceding the Year 8 interview. Again, the majority (80.5%) reported employment; only 27 men (13.2%) said they were employed at any time since Year 1, but not during the preceding year. Of the 165 men who were employed during the preceding year, 22 reported some unemployment within the same year. Thus the categories *employed, unemployed,* and *retired* are somewhat tenuous and shifting, and at times the numbers of men in each category may vary due to the lack of clear distinctions in work status categories.

Before we consider the perceptions, reactions, and experiences of those men employed at Year 8, it should be noted that the occupational composition of the remaining study cohort differed in several ways from the one at intake.[1] As Table 3–2 shows, the group at Year 8 has a markedly higher proportion of upper white-collar workers and, concomitantly, a lower proportion of blue-collar workers than prevailed at the beginning of the study. One of the major reasons for the differences in these distribu-

Table 3-2.   Occupational Status of Cohorts
at Week 7 and Year 8

| | Interview Stage | | | | |
| | Week 7 | | Year 8 | | |
Occupational Status†	Percent	N	Percent	N	Net Difference in Percent
Professional and Managerial	18.3	63	20.6	29	+ 2.3
Upper White Collar	13.3	46	24.8	35	+ 11.5
Lower White Collar	21.4	74	18.4	26	− 3.0
Skilled Blue Collar	18.0	62	14.9	21	− 3.1
Semiskilled and Unskilled Blue Collar	29.0	100	21.3	30	− 7.7
Total	100.0	345	100.0	141*	

*Only patients employed at Year 8 are included in column.
†See Note 1 at end of chapter for description of occupational categories.

tions, as we have seen in Chapter 2, is that the semiskilled and unskilled blue-collar patients suffered significantly higher death rates from heart disease than those in the upper occupational groups. This attrition among these manual workers must be borne in mind as we examine the views and experiences of those workers who are still employed at Year 8.

Perceptions of Work as Causing Heart Disease

There is little question that the heart patients think work is very important in the etiology of their heart attacks. At Week 7, as many as 80% of the patients cited their work as an important factor contributing to their heart attacks, mentioning either emotional tension, physical overwork, or both. At Year 1, these beliefs in the significance of their work as a factor in etiology were held by an even larger percentage (86%) of the heart patients.

We wanted to learn whether this view is still maintained several years after the heart attack. We also wanted to ascertain (1) how occupational groups differ in their perceptions of work as a cause of their myocardial infarctions, and (2) whether severity of illness, or the occurrence of rehospitalizations for heart disease between Year 1 and Year 8, affect the men's perceptions of work as an etiological factor.

As Table 3–3 shows, at Year 8 nearly two-thirds of those men currently employed feel that job-related emotional tension in particular was important in the etiology of their heart attacks. At Year 8, as in previous periods of our study, about half of the heart patients also consider physical exertion to be an important factor in the etiology of their illness.

Considering the employed men as a whole at Year 8, 76% cited either emotional tension and/or physical overwork as factors causing their heart attack. In fact, one-third of the employed men cited *both* factors as relevant to their own cases.

In general, executives, professionals, and white-collar workers are more likely to cite emotional tension as an etiological factor than are the skilled, semiskilled, and unskilled workers. As might be expected, blue-collar workers tend to emphasize the importance of physical exertion more than their white-collar or professional counterparts. These different attributions are

Table 3-3. Perception of the Importance of Work in Etiology of the Heart Attack at Three Points in Time

			Occupational Group			
Interview Stage and Population	Total	Professional and Managerial	White Collar	Skilled Blue Collar	Semiskilled and Unskilled Blue Collar	p*
Percent Reporting Emotional Tension at Work as Important Factor						
Week 7 Total population by pre-illness occupational group	65.2 (221)(339)	76.2 (48)(63)	74.8 (89)(119)	57.4 (35)(61)	51.0 (49)(96)	.001
Year 1 Total population by pre-illness occupational group	74.7 (215)(288)	84.5 (49)(58)	75.0 (72)(96)	76.9 (40)(52)	65.9 (54)(82)	.10*
Year 8 Total population by pre-illness occupational group	68.1 (139)(204)	80.0 (36)(45)	68.5 (50)(73)	60.5 (23)(38)	62.5 (30)(48)	NS
Employed men only by pre-illness occupational group	63.6 (89)(140)	74.3 (26)(35)	65.3 (32)(49)	52.0 (13)(25)	58.1 (18)(31)	NS
Employed men only by current occupational group	63.6 (89)(140)	72.4 (21)(29)	68.3 (41)(60)	71.4 (15)(21)	40.0 (12)(30)	.05

80

Table 3-3 (Continued)

		Occupational Group				
Interview Stage and Population	Total	Professional and Managerial	White Collar	Skilled Blue Collar	Semiskilled and Unskilled Blue Collar	p*
Percent Reporting Physical Exertion at Work as Important Factor						
Week 7						
Total population by pre-illness occupational group	51.7 (172)/(333)	34.4 (21)/(61)	45.0 (54)/(120)	55.9 (33)/(59)	68.8 (64)/(93)	.001
Year 1						
Total population by pre-illness occupational group	51.9 (149)/(287)	37.5 (21)/(56)	43.3 (42)/(97)	58.5 (31)/(53)	67.9 (55)/(81)	.001
Year 8						
Total population by pre-illness occupational group	50.2 (102)/(203)	37.8 (17)/(45)	43.2 (32)/(74)	68.4 (26)/(38)	58.8 (27)/(46)	.02
Employed men only by pre-illness occupational group	47.9 (67)/(140)	31.4 (11)/(35)	46.0 (23)/(50)	72.0 (18)/(25)	50.0 (15)/(30)	.05
Employed men only by current occupational group	47.9 (67)/(140)	31.0 (9)/(29)	41.7 (25)/(60)	76.2 (16)/(21)	56.7 (17)/(30)	.01

*p = level of significance as indicated on the chi-square test. NS = not significant. For a note on reporting of "p" levels greater than .05, see Note 3, Chapter 1.

understandable since professional and white-collar workers report experiencing relatively more emotional stress and less physical exertion, whereas the contrary holds for manual workers. Hence, it would be expected for each group to assign blame to the most distinctive or salient aspects of their work. What is to be emphasized here is the striking consistency over a 7-year period in individual conceptions about etiological factors in their heart disease. Each occupational group remains quite consistent between Year 1 and Year 8 with regard to the importance assigned to work-related tension and physical exertion as causes of their heart attacks. The patterns remain fairly consistent and do not vary with hospitalization or the severity of illness experienced by the patients.

Work Load and Belief in Work Stress as a Factor in Etiology

Despite widespread beliefs among the patients about the etiological role of work stresses in the development of their illness, many of the employed men continued to work long hours at their jobs. In fact, one-fourth of those in the work force at Year 8 reported working 50 to 70 hours a week. Whether or not patients had been rehospitalized over the years made no difference in the high work load pattern: the proportions of those never rehospitalized and those with one or more rehospitalizations because of heart disease were similar among those patients whose work load was heaviest.

However, differences appeared among men from various levels of the occupational scale. Half of the professionals and higher level executives reported working 50 hours or more, and about one-third of small businessmen and lower level executives did so. Among the clerical and blue-collar wage earners the percentages were smaller, averaging 11%.

These data show a marked reduction from the pattern of work load before the first heart attack. For example, in the period before the first hospitalization, fully half of the employed men had worked at least 50 hours each week.[2] Despite the general drop from the time spent at work in the pre-illness period, it is notable that high proportions of the professionals, executives, and small businessmen were still working long hours as of Year 8.

Further, we can note that many of these men at the same time believed that work was an important cause of their heart attack. Yet they nevertheless persisted with their heavy time commitments to their work.

Stresses at Work: Change Over Time

We have seen that heart patients ascribe considerable importance to the pressures of the job in the etiology of their illness. How stressful do they find their jobs over time? At each stage, patients were asked the following questions developed by researchers in the Midtown Manhattan study (Langner & Michael, 1963): "We are interested in how you generally feel at the end of an average day in your regular line of work. Do you often feel pressed for time? Do you often have a feeling of dissatisfaction with your work? Does your work often affect your digestion or sleep, or upset your health in any way? Does your work often stay with you so that you are thinking about it after working hours?"

Table 3–4 presents the responses of different occupational groups to these questions at three points in time.

A number of interesting findings emerge. If we compare data on pre-illness work stress to responses at Year 8, we observe a decrease in reported work stress on almost all items for all population groups over the 8-year period. We should bear in mind, of course, that in reporting on their pre-illness work situation at Week 7, patients may have been prone to overemphasize the amount of stress they may have experienced on the job. Nevertheless, it is important to note that we do not observe a similar uniform decline in all areas of work stress for all groups from Year 1 to Year 8. For example, there is, in fact, a slight increase in reported dissatisfaction with work among white-collar and skilled blue-collar workers during that time. Similarly, for the population as a whole from Year 1 to Year 8, there is an increase in the percentage reporting being pressed for time and feeling that work was adversely affecting their health. Furthermore, as Table 3–4 shows, for all groups but the semiskilled and unskilled, there is an increase in percentages of patients reporting being pressed for time after a day's work.

There is a positive association between occupational status

Table 3-4. Perceptions of Work Stress: Pre-Illness, Year 1, and Year 8*

Reference Point or Interview Stage	Total	Occupational Group[a]				p
		Professional and Managerial	White Collar	Skilled Blue Collar	Semiskilled and Unskilled Blue Collar	
Percent Reporting Frequent Dissatisfaction with Work						
Pre-Illness*	33.7 (115)(341)	35.5 (22)(62)	34.2 (41)(120)	40.0 (24)(60)	28.3 (28)(99)	NS
Year 1	25.1 (61)(243)	32.1 (17)(53)	23.9 (21)(88)	15.2 (7)(46)	28.6 (16)(56)	NS
Year 8	22.7 (32)(141)	27.6 (8)(29)	24.6 (15)(61)	23.8 (5)(21)	13.3 (4)(30)	NS
Percent Reporting Thinking about Work after Hours						
Pre-Illness	50.3 (171)(340)	77.0 (47)(61)	50.8 (61)(120)	46.7 (28)(60)	35.4 (35)(99)	.001
Year 1	37.6 (92)(245)	63.6 (35)(55)	40.9 (36)(88)	23.9 (11)(46)	17.9 (10)(56)	.001
Year 8	35.5 (50)(141)	79.3 (23)(29)	34.4 (21)(61)	14.3 (3)(21)	10.0 (3)(30)	.001

Table 3-4 (Continued)

<table>
<tr><td rowspan="2"></td><td rowspan="2">Reference
Point or
Interview Stage</td><td colspan="6">Occupational Group[†]</td></tr>
<tr><td>Total</td><td>Professional
and Managerial</td><td>White Collar</td><td>Skilled
Blue Collar</td><td>Semiskilled
and Unskilled
Blue Collar</td><td>p</td></tr>
<tr><td rowspan="3">Percent
Reporting
Being
Pressed
for Time</td><td>Pre-Illness</td><td>45.2
(154)
(341)</td><td>59.7
(37)
(62)</td><td>54.2
(65)
(120)</td><td>40.0
(24)
(60)</td><td>28.3
(28)
(99)</td><td>.001</td></tr>
<tr><td>Year 1</td><td>27.6
(67)
(243)</td><td>41.8
(23)
(55)</td><td>28.7
(25)
(87)</td><td>11.1
(5)
(45)</td><td>25.0
(14)
(56)</td><td>.01</td></tr>
<tr><td>Year 8</td><td>31.9
(45)
(141)</td><td>55.2
(16)
(29)</td><td>36.1
(22)
(61)</td><td>19.0
(4)
(21)</td><td>10.0
(3)
(30)</td><td>.001</td></tr>
<tr><td rowspan="3">Percent
Reporting
Work
Affecting
Health</td><td>Pre-Illness</td><td>34.1
(115)
(337)</td><td>41.0
(25)
(61)</td><td>40.7
(48)
(118)</td><td>33.9
(20)
(59)</td><td>22.2
(22)
(99)</td><td>.05</td></tr>
<tr><td>Year 1</td><td>16.4
(40)
(244)</td><td>24.1
(13)
(54)</td><td>20.5
(18)
(88)</td><td>6.5
(3)
(46)</td><td>10.7
(6)
(56)</td><td>.C5</td></tr>
<tr><td>Year 8</td><td>19.3
(27)
(140)</td><td>24.1
(7)
(29)</td><td>26.7
(16)
(60)</td><td>14.3
(3)
(21)</td><td>3.3
(1)
(30)</td><td>.10</td></tr>
</table>

*Responses concerning the pre-illness period were gathered at Week 7. Cohorts include only those currently employed at time of interview.

[†]Patients are categorized by pre-illness occupational group at the first two stages and by current occupation at Year 8.

85

and reported work stress on all items but one—frequent dissatisfaction with work. One conspicuous and consistent finding is that in comparison with other patients, those in the upper occupational categories report experiencing greater work stress on each of the other three items at Week 7, at Year 1 and at Year 8. It should be noted, too, that at Year 8, almost four-fifths of the professionals and managerial workers report thinking about work after hours, and that more than one-half of them report being pressed for time. Indeed, the percentage of professionals and managerial workers who report thinking about work after hours actually rises slightly from Week 7 to Year 8—a dramatic exception to the general decline in work stress during the total period.

It is possible that over time, semiskilled and unskilled patients, in particular (who even prior to their illness showed less involvement in their work), are able to adjust to their illness or to defend themselves psychologically by becoming even less emotionally invested in their jobs. Hence, they may find their work less stressful. Our data also suggest that other heart patients, especially professionals and managerial workers, may find it more difficult or undesirable to appreciably lower their threshold of job involvement and accompanying job stress. It is also possible that some of the findings we have observed may be attributed to changes in the composition of the study population. Thus, ostensible changes within occupational groups may be due to differential attrition from the work force over time. None of these findings, however, are related to differential severity of illness.

Physical Activity at Work

Table 3–5 reports on the prevalence of on-the-job lifting, sitting, and walking for different occupational groups. As we would expect, there are marked differences between the heart patients who are professional or managerial and those in other occupations in the amount of time they spend sitting or walking on the job. As Table 3–5 shows, at all stages—pre-illness, Year 1 and Year 8—a much greater percentage of professionals and managers, as compared with those in other occupations, report sitting at least 50% of the time on the job. Conversely, most manual workers spend more than 50% of their time walking on the job, a finding that also holds at all three points that are measured in the study. It would appear that the heart patients do not have much leeway in modifying the amount of sitting or walking they do in a given job.

Our findings suggest, however, that heart patients, particularly manual workers, have some flexibility in amount of lifting they do on the job. Semiskilled and unskilled workers did substantially less lifting at Year 1 than before their heart attacks, and at Year 8 the reported lifting in this group was similar to that at Year 1. Thus, over the long term, it appears that the initial marked reduction in lifting after the heart attack was maintained among the semiskilled and unskilled patients. As we have seen, the majority of blue-collar workers perceived physical exertion at work as a hazard to their well-being, and the reduction in lifting by the semiskilled and unskilled may be evidence of a deliberate response to the perception of dangers to their health at work.[3]

Problems at Work

One important question relates to the extent to which the patient's heart condition caused problems for him at work. At Week 7 almost half of the patients anticipated overall negative effects on their work. By Year 8 about a third of the patients felt that their health status, in fact, had hurt their work situation. While this represents an improvement, the picture is hardly salutary in absolute terms. Moreover, a higher percentage of heart patients at Year 1 and Year 8 felt that their heart condition had negative effects on their earnings compared with their anticipations at Week 7. Almost one-third of employed workers at Year 8 felt that their earnings had suffered as a result of their illness.

Slightly more (27.5%) of the employed men at Year 8 believed that they experienced negative effects or opportunities for advancement as compared with the expectations of the cohort at Week 7 (20.1%). A considerable percentage of the professional and managerial group (41.4%) at Year 8 thought their opportunities for promotion had suffered. On the other hand, by Year 8 less than one-fifth of the employed semiskilled or unskilled work-

Table 3-5. Physical Activity at Work: Pre-Illness, Year 1, and Year 8*

Reference Point or Interview Stage	Occupational Group†					p
	Total	Professional and Managerial	White Collar	Skilled Blue Collar	Semiskilled and Unskilled Blue Collar	
Percent Reporting Frequent Lifting						
Pre-Illness	32.5 (78/240)	9.3 (4/43)	26.2 (22/84)	32.6 (14/43)	54.3 (38/70)	.001
Year 1	8.2 (20/245)	3.6 (2/55)	6.8 (6/88)	6.5 (3/46)	16.1 (9/56)	--§
Year 8	10.6 (15/141)	0.0 (0/29)	6.6 (4/61)	23.8 (5/21)	20.0 (6/30)	--§
Percent Sitting 50% or More of Time on Job						
Pre-Illness	37.5 (90/240)	76.7 (33/43)	42.9 (36/84)	18.6 (8/43)	18.6 (13/70)	.001
Year 1	54.7 (134/245)	74.5 (41/55)	52.3 (46/88)	47.8 (22/46)	44.6 (25/56)	.01
Year 8	45.4 (64/141)	75.9 (22/29)	45.9 (28/61)	23.8 (5/21)	30.0 (9/30)	.001

Table 3-5 (Continued)

		Occupational Group[†]				
Reference Point or Interview Stage	Total	Professional and Managerial	White Collar	Skilled Blue Collar	Semiskilled and Unskilled Blue Collar	p
Percent Walking 50% or More of Time on Job[#]						
Pre-Illness	55.4 (133)/(240)	34.9 (15)/(43)	56.0 (47)/(84)	58.1 (25)/(43)	65.8 (46)/(70)	.02
Year 1	50.6 (124)/(245)	34.5 (19)/(55)	55.7 (49)/(88)	52.2 (24)/(46)	57.1 (32)/(56)	.10
Year 8	53.9 (76)/(141)	20.7 (6)/(29)	54.1 (33)/(61)	66.7 (14)/(21)	76.7 (23)/(30)	.001

*Responses concerning the pre-illness period were gathered at Week 7. Cohorts include only those currently employed at time of interview.

†Patients are categorized by pre-illness occupational group at the first two time points (Pre-illness, Year 1) and by current occupation at Year 8.

#Because these items were added after the interview program had begun, Week 7 responses are available for 240 men, or 70 percent of the total cohort at that time.

§Chi-square values were not computed because of small numbers in cells.

ers felt similarly. It is possible that the latter finding may be attributable to lower levels of expectations among workers in the lowest occupational category.

Of particular interest, however, is the fact that those who had been rehospitalized for heart disease from Year 1 to Year 8 were more likely to report experiencing problems at work. Thirty-six percent of those who had been rehospitalized for their heart conditions indicated that they had problems at work related to their illness as compared with only 16% of those who had not been rehospitalized and only 5% of those who had been rehospitalized for nonheart conditions. Moreover, those rehospitalized for heart conditions were more likely to perceive their chances for promotion and long-term advancement to have been negatively affected. As many as 43% of those who were rehospitalized for their heart conditions experienced negative effects relating to promotion and advancement as compared with only 24% of those who had not been rehospitalized and 16% who had been hospitalized for reasons other than heart disease.

Patients were also asked at Week 7 and at Year 1 whether their heart condition affected their relationships with either their employers or with their fellow workers. At Year 8 we asked separate questions concerning relationships with employers and with co-workers. Because of the differences in the questions, we are not able to compare the Year 1 and Year 8 responses directly. However, there appears to be an increase in the reporting of negative effects in relationships with employers (see Table 3–6). At Year 1 approximately 13% of the employed population reported that their illness had handicapped relationships with either employers or with their co-workers. At Year 8, one-quarter of employed patients perceived negative effects on their relationships with employers, and about 9% felt that their relationship with fellow workers had suffered because of their illness.

FINANCES

Financial resources also constitute one of the key elements in the patient's "armory of resources."[4] Patients with sufficient funds are obviously more equipped to cope with the material if

Table 3-6. Effects of Heart Attack on Work: Patients' Predictions (Week 7) and Reported Experiences (Year 1 and Year 8)

		Occupational Group				
Interview Stage and Population	Total*	Professional and Managerial	White Collar	Skilled Blue Collar	Semiskilled and Unskilled Blue Collar	p
Percent Perceiving Effects on Work						
Week 7 Total population by pre-illness occupational group	46.3 (132)/(285)	37.5 (21)/(56)	39.4 (41)/(104)	50.0 (22)/(44)	59.3 (48)/(81)	.02
Year 1 Employed men only by pre-illness occupational group	44.9 (123)/(274)	37.9 (22)/(58)	38.9 (37)/(95)	44.0 (22)/(50)	59.2 (42)/(71)	.05
Year 8 Total population by pre-illness occupational group	35.6 (68)/(191)	43.2 (19)/(44)	29.2 (21)/(72)	38.2 (13)/(34)	36.6 (15)/(41)	NS
Employed men only by pre-illness occupational group	33.6 (47)/(140)	42.9 (15)/(35)	30.0 (15)/(50)	33.3 (8)/(24)	29.0 (9)/(31)	NS
Employed men only by current occupational group	33.6 (47)/(140)	34.5 (10)/(29)	37.7 (23)/(61)	20.0 (4)/(20)	33.3 (10)/(30)	NS

Table 3-6 (Continued)

| | | Occupational Group | | | | |
Interview Stage and Population	Total*	Professional and Managerial	White Collar	Skilled Blue Collar	Semiskilled and Unskilled Blue Collar	p
Percent Perceiving Negative Effects on Promotion or Opportunities for Advancement						
Week 7 — Total population by pre-illness occupational group	20.1 (55) (273)	11.1 (5) (45)	18.6 (18) (97)	20.8 (10) (48)	26.5 (22) (83)	NS
Year 1 — Employed men only by pre-illness occupational group	29.8 (71) (238)	29.2 (14) (48)	28.6 (24) (84)	25.0 (11) (44)	35.5 (22) (62)	NS
Year 8 — Total population by pre-illness occupational group	30.2 (57) (189)	41.9 (18) (43)	22.2 (16) (72)	38.2 (13) (34)	25.0 (10) (40)	NS
Employed men only by pre-illness occupational group	27.5 (38) (138)	41.2 (14) (34)	22.0 (11) (50)	33.3 (8) (24)	16.7 (5) (30)	NS
Employed men only by current occupational group	27.5 (38) (138)	41.4 (12) (29)	23.4 (14) (60)	33.3 (7) (21)	17.9 (5) (28)	NS

Table 3-6 (Continued)

		Occupational Group				
Interview Stage and Population	Total*	Professional and Managerial	White Collar	Skilled Blue Collar	Semiskilled and Unskilled Blue Collar	p
Percent Perceiving Negative Effects on Earnings						
Week 7						
Total population by pre-illness occupational group	23.3 (68/292)	26.9 (14/52)	20.0 (22/110)	19.2 (10/52)	28.2 (22/78)	NS
Year 1						
Employed men only by pre-illness occupational group	36.5 (99/271)	26.3 (15/57)	28.3 (26/92)	42.3 (22/52)	51.4 (36/70)	.01
Year 8						
Total population by pre-illness occupational group	32.1 (61/190)	36.4 (16/44)	29.6 (21/71)	37.1 (13/35)	27.5 (11/40)	NS
Employed men only by pre-illness occupational group	29.3 (41/140)	34.3 (12/35)	26.0 (13/50)	36.0 (9/25)	23.3 (7/30)	NS
Employed men only by current occupational group	29.3 (41/140)	27.6 (8/29)	34.4 (21/61)	20.0 (4/20)	26.7 (8/30)	NS

93

Table 3-6 (Continued)

	Interview Stage and Population	Occupational Group					
		Total*	Professional and Managerial	White Collar	Skilled Blue Collar	Semiskilled and Unskilled Blue Collar	p
Percent Perceiving Effects on Relationships with Employer or Co-Workers	**Week 7** Total population by pre-illness occupational group	16.3 (48)(294)	12.0 (6)(50)	10.0 (10)(100)	17.6 (9)(51)	24.7 (23)(93)	.05
	Year 1 Employed men only by pre-illness occupational group	12.9 (30)(233)	16.0 (8)(50)	9.5 (8)(84)	6.5 (3)(46)	20.8 (11)(53)	.20
Percent Perceiving Effects on Relationships with Employer	**Year 8** Total population by pre-illness occupational group	25.1 (43)(171)	29.7 (11)(37)	26.7 (16)(60)	23.5 (8)(34)	20.0 (8)(40)	NS
	Employed men only by pre-illness occupational group	25.2 (32)(127)	30.0 (9)(30)	26.2 (11)(42)	29.2 (7)(24)	16.1 (5)(31)	NS
	Employed men only by current occupational group	25.2 (32)(127)	22.7 (5)(22)	31.5 (17)(54)	19.0 (4)(21)	20.0 (6)(30)	NS

Table 3-6 (Continued)

Interview Stage and Population	Total*		Professional and Managerial	White Collar	Skilled Blue Collar	Semiskilled and Unskilled Blue Collar	p
		Occupational Group					
Percent Perceiving Effects on Relationships with Co-Workers							
<u>Year 8</u>							
Total population by pre-illness occupational group	6.9 (13)(189)		4.8 (2)(42)	8.6 (6)(70)	11.8 (4)(34)	2.4 (1)(41)	--†
Employed men only by pre-illness occupational group	8.6 (12)(139)		5.7 (2)(35)	10.2 (5)(49)	16.7 (4)(24)	3.2 (1)(31)	--†
Employed men only by current occupational group	8.6 (12)(139)		3.4 (1)(29)	8.5 (5)(59)	14.3 (3)(21)	10.0 (3)(30)	--†

*"Don't Know" and "No Response" categories have been excluded. Because of the difference in the numbers of patients answering each question, the "N's" are reported in parentheses underneath the percentages.

†Chi-square values were not computed because of small numbers in cells.

not the emotional costs of illness. Even if the patient has available financial resources at the beginning of his illness, these may be depleted over time, especially when the condition is chronic. In addition, we will examine whether the illness also had negative effects on the financial circumstances of the patient's family. For these reasons, then, we examine how the heart patients fared financially at Year 8, as compared with Year 1.

In reviewing patients' financial situations and the costs of illness at Year 1, we found several downward changes in earnings. Those who were rehospitalized suffered the greatest degree of salary loss and the sharpest decline in total family income. Out-of-pocket costs of care were directly related to occupational status, those in the higher brackets incurring the highest out-of-pocket expenses.[5] During the first year, the lower income groups initiated greater changes in their spending patterns than groups with higher incomes. Those who reported significant problems during the first year most often cited the areas of finances and work. Blue-collar workers experienced the most difficulty. We should bear these findings in mind as we look at the heart patient population at Year 8. What, then, are their financial circumstances 8 years after their first heart attacks, at an average age of 59?

Financial Status at Year 8

As we have noted, 63% of the surviving patients were employed full time, and approximately 5% part time at Year 8. About 31% were out of the work force, 25% due to retirement and 6% to unemployment. This represents a marked increase over Year 1 in the proportion of subjects who were retired, as would be expected in a study group of whom nearly one-fifth had passed their sixty-fifth birthday by their final interview.

Sources of Income at Year 8.   Many patients reported more than one source of income. Approximately 71% earned some income from their own wages or salaries. Forty-eight percent obtained some income from the wages of other family members. Sixteen percent derived income from self-employment or independent business activities. Approximately 14% received some income from rental property.

Additional income as derived from various forms of social insurance and pension plans. Fifteen percent received some income from Social Security retirement benefits, and 10% from Social Security disability benefits. Sixteen percent of the subjects reported receiving some income from veterans' benefits, and 14% from private employer or union benefits. As Table 3–7 indicates, a few patients received benefits from other sources as well.

Comparing the populations at Year 1 and Year 8, we find increased reliance on governmental sources of assistance, particularly Social Security retirement benefits and Social Security disability benefits. Assistance from the Veterans Administration increased from 2% at Year 1 to 16% at Year 8. Like the general population, then, these heart patients rely increasingly on government financial assistance as they grow older.

Patients' Attitudes Toward Social Security Payments

Of the 46 men who reported receiving Social Security payments at Year 8, two-thirds ($N = 31$) characterized the payments as inadequate. Among these 31 recipients, 30 expressed

Table 3-7. Principal Sources of Income at Year 8

Source of Income	Number of Patients (N = 205)	Percent*
Own wages or salary	145	70.7
Wages of other family member	98	47.8
Own business income (self-employed)	32	15.6
Rental income	28	13.7
Institutional and organizational sources		
Social Security retirement benefits	30	14.6
Social Security disability benefits	21	10.2
Veterans benefits	32	15.6
Private employer or union benefits	28	13.7
Unemployment Compensation	13	6.4
Private insurance disability benefits	12	5.9
Public assistance (welfare)	6	3.0
Worker's Compensation	3	1.5
Supplemental Security Income (SSI)	2	1.0
Private insurance retirement benefits	1	.5

*Percentages are not cumulative as some patients reported multiple sources of income.

the view that the benefits did not provide enough money to live on. Surprisingly, those rehospitalized and those not rehospitalized reported in equal proportions that Social Security funds were not enough to live on. In evaluating these findings, we should keep in mind the purposes of the Social Security program itself. The program was not initially designed to serve as a sole source of income, but rather as a supplement to other personal resources.

Income Loss From Work at Year 1 and Year 8

With regard to the amount of income lost from work in the previous year because of ill health, the results are very different in the eighth year, as compared with the first year. At Year 1, as many as 50% of the patients reported some loss of income from work as a result of their illness. Table 3–8 shows that the results are strikingly different at Year 8, and, indeed, surprisingly more favorable, when only 10% of those who had worked during the preceding year indicated they had lost income due to illness during that time. In other words, 90% of those employed at any time in the foregoing year experienced no loss of income from work because of ill health.[6] Of those employed men who had been rehospitalized during the preceding year ($N = 16$), only three reported lost income due to illness.

Table 3-8.   Reported Loss of Income from Work
in Preceding Year Due to Ill Health

	Percent of Total Year 8 Population	Percent of Patients in Work Force During Year	Number of Patients
Lost Income from Work	7.8	9.8	16
No Lost Income from Work	72.2	90.2	148
Not in Work Force During Past Year	20.0	--	41
Total	100.0	100.0	205

Among the men who reported a loss of income from illness in the preceding year, the amounts were relatively low. For example, of the 16 patients shown in Table 3–8 with loss of income, 6 reported the loss was $600 or less. At the upper extreme, four men reported $6000 or more as the amount lost. Since the small number of men reporting income loss did not permit a breakdown by occupation, it was impossible to ascertain whether manual workers differed from white-collar workers in severity of income loss.

In interpreting these apparently favorable results about the limited effect of illness on income loss at Year 8, which contrast markedly with findings at Year 1, we should remember that the population at Year 8 differs from that at Year 1 in two main respects. First, an appreciable number of patients died during the 7-year period. Moreover, a significantly higher proportion of deaths in the interim occurred among semiskilled and unskilled workers, a group normally more vulnerable economically to the effects of illness. At Year 1 as many as three-quarters of the semiskilled and unskilled men suffered some loss of income from work because of illness, more than any other occupational group. Second, as we have seen, almost a third of the patients had left the labor force because of retirement or unemployment. Accordingly, the relatively small reported loss of income may be largely explained by the fact that those who might be most vulnerable to loss of income at work were able to make use of Social Security, disability, or other insurance benefits.

The Costs of Illness

Personal Costs of Illness: Year 1 and Year 8.   The pattern of estimated out-of-pocket or personal costs of illness in the eighth year is fairly similar to that in the first year (Table 3–9), although figures have not been adjusted for inflation. For example, 31% of the respondents in the first year and 27% in the eighth year reported no expenditures for medicines. Approximately 55% of the population at Year 1 and 62% at Year 8 reported no costs for laboratory tests. Approximately one-third of the patients reported no expenditures for doctors' bills in the first year; in the eighth year, virtually the same proportion reported no costs for doctors' bills.

Table 3-9. Out-of-Pocket Costs of Illness During Preceding Year
at Year 1 and Year 8: By Patient Reports

Year 1 (N = 293)

Out-of-Pocket Costs by Percent of Year 1 Population[*]

Item	None	$1-99	$100-199	$200-399	$400-599	$600 or more	NR[†]
Medicines	31.5	41.2	15.0	9.2	--	--	3.1
Laboratory tests	54.9	28.6	10.2	2.1	--	--	4.2
Physicians' services	34.5	31.4	10.6	5.4	1.4	.7	16.0

Year 8 (N = 205)

Out-of-Pocket Costs by Percent of Year 8 Population[*]

Item	None	$1-99	$100-149	$150-249	$250 or more	NR[†]
Medicines	27.3	43.5	11.7	7.3	9.8	.4
Laboratory tests	62.4	27.8	5.4	2.0	2.0	.4

	None	$1-99	$100-199	$200-399	$400-or more	NR[†]
Physicians' services	33.2	43.9	11.2	10.7 [§]	--	1.0
Total cost of illness reported[‡]	15.6	30.7	24.0	18.5	11.2	--

[*]Figures are not adjusted for inflation.

[†]NR includes "no response," "don't know," and uncodable responses.

[‡]Reported total cost includes medicine, laboratory tests, and physicians' services only.

[§]Coding category for this item is "$200 or more."

100

Rehospitalization and Costs of Care at Year 8.   As we saw, approximately 35% of the Year 8 population had been rehospitalized since Year 1 for heart-related problems; an additional 28% were rehospitalized for noncardiac problems, and a little over one-third (approximately 37%) had not been rehospitalized since Year 1.

Nearly all members of the study population had health insurance of some kind. Accordingly, many of the expenses they incurred were covered by insurance. It is hardly surprising that the sickest patients—those rehospitalized for their heart conditions or other ailments—consistently spent the most on medical and other health-related expenditures. For example, 29% of the nonrehospitalized patients reported no out-of-pocket expenditures for medicine in contrast to only 14% of the recently heart-rehospitalized patients. About 27% of the heart-rehospitalized group reported yearly out-of-pocket payments for medicine exceeding $150; only 12% of the nonrehospitalized report comparable expenses.

For laboratory tests and electrocardiograms, 14% of the heart-rehospitalized group and only 4% of the nonrehospitalized group reported payments exceeding $100. Thirty-three percent of the heart-rehospitalized men spent over $100 of personal funds on doctor bills; only 16% of the nonrehospitalized men did so. Over 10% of the heart-rehospitalized group spent $300 or more in the past year for hospital or nursing care, which was not reimbursed. Are the problems of the heart patient being exacerbated by the additional burdens of health care expenses that are not covered by insurance? Although these differences are not of statistical significance, the finding that a larger proportion of those rehospitalized for heart disease suffer substantial personal nonreimbursed financial costs may merit concern and may require more intensive study for policy formulation.

The Financial Impact of Illness: Life Changes and Problems at Year 8. At Year 8, patients were asked the following open-ended question: "Thinking back over the past few years, in what ways has illness changed your life?" Although 78% of the men indicated that illness had changed their lives in at least one major way, surprisingly, only 7% reported that their illness had created or intensified financial problems. Change in activity level was mentioned by a far greater proportion of patients (44%).

Nor did the patients' illness appear to have much influence on their wives' employment status. At Year 8, 54% of wives were employed, a figure consistent with data on women in the work force of the United States as a whole (Booth, 1973). Only 14% of all husbands reported that the illness strongly affected their wives' decisions to work at this time. These data are analogous to findings which emerged at Year 1. At that time, about half of the wives were employed, and 4% of married men cited their illness as an influential factor.

Asked what had been their biggest problems during the past year, only 16% of the patients named financial problems; finances, however, were the most frequently cited problem. In response to the question, "Considering your total situation at present, what do you see as your biggest concerns or problems for the future?," financial problems were cited by one-fifth of the men, second only to survival and health concerns. This finding is consistent with the pattern of response to a similar question dealing with anticipated problems at Year 1.

Finances may be an even more important problem for heart patients than our data indicate. For one thing, predominant worries about health, activity level, and survival may override perceived financial concerns and mute their salience. As we have seen, almost one-third of the patients are retired or unemployed and most of them testify in response to other questions that Social Security benefits are insufficient for their needs. Most of the men are older and by Year 8 have been coping with their heart conditions for an extended period of time, and probably have been lowering their level of expectations.

SUMMARY

Eight years after their first myocardial infarctions, most of the heart patients in the study population were gainfully employed. A majority reported at Year 8 that they had worked at least part of the time since Year 1. Almost one-third of the surviving heart patients were no longer in the work force at Year 8, and over 60% of these had left for reasons related to health.

Two-thirds or more of the patients at Week 7, Year 1 and

Year 8 cited work tension as a major contributing factor to their illness. Neither severity of illness nor rehospitalization for heart disease was significantly related to the perception of work as an important factor in etiology. Patients in the upper occupational categories reported more work-related stress than lower level workers. Heart patients decreased the amount of on-the-job lifting they did prior to their illness.

Men who were rehospitalized for heart conditions were most likely to encounter problems at work. Almost twice as many men who were rehospitalized for heart conditions experienced problems relating to promotion and advancement, compared with those who were not rehospitalized.

At the time of the Year 8 interview, nearly three-quarters of the men were receiving some income from wages or salary. A high proportion of the retired men received Social Security benefits, and reliance on social insurance and pension plans had increased since Year 1. Two-thirds of the men receiving Social Security payments at Year 8 described the benefits as inadequate.

The pattern of loss of income from work differed markedly at Year 1 and Year 8. At Year 1, approximately 50% of the employed men reported loss of income from work in the preceding year due to illness-related problems; at Year 8 the comparable figure was only 10%.

Asked about their major concerns for the future, one-fifth mentioned finances. While most patients in the study population faced relatively few work-related problems due to their illness, a sizeable proportion encountered difficulties and disadvantages. It would seem that an appreciable number of heart patients may require various forms of guidance and assistance such as financial supplements, job training, counseling, and special arrangements so that they are not subject to additional penalties which may exacerbate their conditions.

NOTES

1. In classifying patients by occupational status at Year 8, we have used the following five categories:

    1. Professionals, managers, and proprietors of medium-sized and large businesses.

2. Upper white-collar workers, including administrative personnel of large concerns, owners of small independent businesses, and semi-professionals.

3. Lower white-collar workers, including clerical and sales workers and technicians.

4. Skilled blue-collar workers.

5. Semiskilled and unskilled blue-collar workers.

In our earlier work, *The Heart Patient Recovers,* a four-point occupational status classification was used, in which categories 2 and 3 (upper and lower white-collar workers) were combined into a single white-collar category.

The categories combined are analogous to occupational categories 3 and 4 in the Hollingshead Index of Social Position (1957). For purposes of comparison of Year 8 materials with earlier data, various tables in this chapter employ a four-category system.

2. In the absence of a noncardiac comparison group, we may posit that the reduction in hours worked by blue-collar men may be due in part to a change in the economy. The recession in New England in recent years during the period of the study, for example, may account for less paid overtime for blue-collar workers.

3. It should be pointed out, however, that the attribution of risk to physical exertion remains a complex issue which still requires resolution by empirical research. Epidemiologic data suggest that regular physical activity has beneficial effects on cardiovascular fitness (NHLBI, 1978, pp. 3–7), hence, the exact ways in which physical activity on the job affects cardiovascular health require further assessment.

4. For reviews of the major costs of cardiac illness in both direct and indirect terms, see, for example, Klarman, 1965; Mushkin and Collings, 1959; Rice, 1965, 1966; and Smith and Lilienfeld, 1971.

5. We can note that this finding obtains for the general population, as well. However, it should also be noted that out-of-pocket expenses may comprise a greater proportion of the total financial resources of the lower income groups (Andersen, Lion, & Anderson, 1976, pp. 134–5).

6. Twenty percent of the patients had not been employed at all during the preceding year.

Chapter 4

USE OF SERVICES AND SUPPORTIVE PROGRAMS

Health care policy makers, administrators, and students of the health delivery system have expressed growing interest in the access which people have to a range of health services and supportive programs (Aday & Andersen, 1975; Aday & Eichhorn, 1972; Andersen, Lion, & Anderson, 1976; Anderson & Andersen, 1972; Bice & White, 1971; Donabedian, 1972; Kahn, 1973). While writers have given increasing attention to escalating costs, they have also been concerned with availability of different services and the factors that affect their use. For heart patients in this study, there were a wide variety of health professionals, agencies, institutions, and care facilities, as well as social service organizations and personnel whose help they could seek. Although all these resources were available, and constituted possible resources for the patient, some were used considerably while relatively little use was made of others.

Use of Physicians

A most conspicuous finding about patients' use of services at Year 8 is very high reliance on physicians, who understandably serve as the mainstay of health care for heart patients. This pattern of high physician use is consistent with findings at Year 1.

Almost 90% ($N = 183$) of the patients reporting at Year 8 said they had seen a doctor in the foregoing year. Of these, over half ($N = 96$) reported having seen more than one physician; one-fifth ($N = 38$) reported visiting at least three physicians. Only a small minority, 22 patients, had not seen a physician within the preceding year. The patients in our study use physicians' services at a higher rate than that reported in studies of the general population (Andersen, Lion, & Anderson, 1976, p. 44).

The patient-physician relationship tends to be both established and enduring. Most visits to physicians are not prompted by symptoms of acute illness or discomfort due to heart conditions or other ailments. Instead, over half ($N = 94$) the patients who had seen doctors reported doing so mainly for routine examinations or periodic checkups. Of those who did visit their physicians because of illness, 58% ($N = 51$) indicated that the illness was not heart related. Thus approximately three-quarters of those who had seen a physician during the preceding year did so as a regular procedure or for illness unrelated to their heart condition. Although this finding attests to the routinization and acceptance of the doctor-patient relationship, it may merit some qualification. The participants' special status as heart patients may prompt an appreciable number of them to value the routine examination as a means of ruling out any disturbing symptoms and obtaining reassurance that they are progressing well.

Approximately four-fifths ($N = 162$) of the patients at Year 8 had seen a private physician, as opposed to a clinic physician or no physician. Moreover, about three-quarters ($N = 149$) reported having a regular doctor for the care of their hearts. It appears that the patients in general place high value on having the same physician over time. Indeed, 96% of the patients who had a regular doctor to care for their heart conditions reported that they planned to continue seeing the same doctor.

Furthermore, fully 62% of the patients had the same regular physicians at Year 8 as at Year 1. This record of continuity over a 7-year period underlines the stability of the doctor-patient relationship and most patients' apparent satisfaction with this relationship. Of those patients who changed physicians most moved in the direction of more specialized care. Three-quarters of those who changed turned to an internist or cardiologist for care.

Use of Clinics, Emergency Rooms, and Other Outpatient Facilities

Although the private physician was the predominant source of care, two-fifths of the patients ($N = 80$) reported that in the preceding year they had obtained at least some medical care in a clinic, emergency room, or other outpatient facility (see Table 4–1). Almost one-fifth of the patients made use of such facilities more than once during the foregoing year. Thirty percent made use of such services in addition to care provided by their regular physicians. The extent to which the use of clinics may reflect dissatisfaction with the private physician is unclear from the data.

Use of Inpatient Hospital Services

In our earlier study, we observed that approximately one-fifth of the patients were rehospitalized within the first year following their heart attacks, and that a considerable number experienced heart-related symptoms. Although the picture

Table 4-1. Visits to Clinics, Emergency Rooms, and Outpatient Facilities in Preceding Year: For Heart-Related Conditions

Total Number of Visits	Percent of Total Year 8 Patients	Number of Patients ($N = 205$)
1	22.0	45
2–5	8.3	17
6–10	4.9	10
11–15	2.4	5
16–20	0	0
21 or more	1.5	3
Subtotal	39.1	80
None	60.9	125
Total	100.0	205

appeared bright by a number of criteria, such as survival and performance of occupational and familial roles, we observed that the patient with heart disease suffers from an ongoing chronic illness that requires frequent and intensive professional services.

Reviewing the data on patients surviving to Year 8, use of inpatient hospital services since Year 1 tends to substantiate our original assessment. Utilization of inpatient hospital services was high: 63% ($N = 130$) of the Year 8 population reported at least one hospitalization since Year 1. Fifty-eight percent ($N = 76$) had been hospitalized more than once during this period, and 17% ($N = 22$) four or more times. Over half of those hospitalized reported at least one heart-related hospitalization, and 42% of these ($N = 30$), reported they were hospitalized for a subsequent heart attack.

Over a quarter ($N = 37$) of the patients hospitalized since Year 1 had been hospitalized within the year prior to the Year 8 interview; about half ($N = 66$) had been hospitalized within the past 2 years. Seventeen men reported that their most recent hospitalizations had occurred over 5 years earlier. Of those patients who reported hospitalizations unrelated to their hearts, 17% ($N = 15$) had been hospitalized within the past year. In contrast, 34% ($N = 24$) of those who reported heart-related hospitalizations had been hospitalized within the past year.[1]

Use of Other Health Professionals and Agencies

Although use of physicians is frequent and well established among these heart patients, it is strikingly evident that they make minimal use of other professionals (see Table 4-2). Ninety-one percent ($N = 186$) reported that they had not received any instructions or advice on health care during the previous year from social workers, dieticians, visiting nurses, chiropractors, or osteopaths. Of these professionals, dieticians were most frequently consulted; this pattern is probably attributable to some patients' concern about weight problems and need for special diets low in cholesterol, lipids, or salt.

Considering the wide range of problems experienced by heart patients, and the kinds of services they could use to advantage, it may be surprising that they make so little use of profes-

Table 4-2. Use of Services of Non-Physician Professionals
in Preceding Year: For Heart-Related Conditions

Professional	Percent and Number of Year 8 Population Reporting Use of Services (Base N = 205)	Number of Visits Reported by Percent of Year 8 Population				
		1	2	3	4	5 +
Dietician	6.8 (14)	4.9 (10)	1.5 (3)			.5 (1)
Visiting Nurse	1.5 (3)	1.0 (2)				.5 (1)
Social Worker	1.0 (2)	.5 (1)				.5 (1)
Osteopath	.5 (1)				.5 (1)	
Chiropractor	0 (0)					

sionals and agencies other than physicians. Patients were asked at
Year 8 whether they had contacted any of a list of agencies and
professionals for help or advice with problems resulting from
their heart conditions since Year 1. As Table 4-3 shows, outpatient hospital services were used by the greatest number of patients over the 7 years: 15% reported contact with outpatient
hospital services between Year 1 and Year 8, and 10% during the
preceding year. Use of outpatient services may have occurred in
conjunction with hospitalizations.

The second most frequently used agency was the unemploy-

Table 4-3.   Distribution of Agencies and Professionals Contacted
for Heart-Related Problems: By Percent of
Year 8 Study Population
Base N = 205

Agency or Professional	Percent and Number Reporting Contact in Year 1 - Year 8 Period	Percent and Number Reporting Contact in Preceding Year
Outpatient hospital services	15.1 (31)	10.2 (21)
Unemployment service	12.2 (25)	4.4 (9)
Veterans Administration	8.8 (18)	3.4 (7)
Psychiatrist	4.4 (9)	1.5 (3)
American Heart Association	2.9 (6)	1.0 (2)
Welfare department	2.9 (6)	.5 (1)
Clergy	2.9 (6)	2.0 (4)
Employment counselor	2.9 (6)	1.0 (2)
Social worker	2.4 (5)	1.5 (3)
Cardiac rehabilitation clinic	2.4 (5)	2.0 (4)
Visiting Nurse Association	2.0 (4)	2.0 (4)
Group therapist	2.0 (4)	1.5 (3)
Marriage counselor	1.0 (2)	1.0 (2)
Social service agency, such as Family Service Association	1.0 (2)	.5 (1)
Other	4.4 (9)	1.5 (3)

ment service, consulted by 12% of the patients ($N = 25$) between Year 1 and Year 8. Use of this resource probably reflected employment problems experienced by some patients, which were apparent at Year 1. The Veterans Administration ranked third with 9%. No other agency or professional had been contacted by more than 5% of the population. Furthermore, almost two-thirds ($N = 130$) of the patients reported that they had not had contact with *any* of the listed agencies or professionals. Of the 74 patients who reported contacting any of the agencies listed in Table 4-3, three-quarters had used only one. This low utilization rate for these health and social services is consistent with our observations at Year 1 (see Table 4-4).

Many complex factors underlie this pattern of comparatively low use of important agencies, professionals, and institutions in the community by these heart patients. This low usage could be attributable to such factors as lack of knowledge or appreciation on the part of attending physicians of the services provided by these professionals and agencies, lack of interest or willingness by patients to use these services, inaccessibility or unresponsiveness by these agencies or professionals, or that they may not provide

Table 4-4. Distribution of Institutional and Professional
Contacts Most Frequently Mentioned at Year 1

Agency or Professional	Percent of Total Year 1 Population	Number of Patients (Base $N = 293$)
Unemployment service	11.3	33
Welfare department	6.6	19
Clergy	5.5	16
Veterans Administration	4.4	13
American Heart Association	4.1	12
Social worker	4.1	12
Cardiac rehabilitation clinic	2.7	8
Social service agency	1.7	5
Psychiatrist	.6	2
Visiting Nurse Association	.3	1

those particular services that heart patients need or deem to be necessary. Although our emphasis in collecting the data was on the patterns themselves rather than the various underlying causal factors, the basis for these results deserves further exploration and assessment.

Social Security: A High-Usage Benefit

Patients were also asked whether they had ever applied for assistance from any of the following predominantly financial benefits: Worker's Compensation, veterans' benefits, private insurance disability payments, public assistance (welfare), or Social Security. Patients who reported applying for a particular program were questioned about receipt of aid during the previous year. Responses are presented in Table 4-5.

Over a quarter of the Year 8 population had applied for Social Security benefits at some time in their lives, making it the most heavily utilized resource of the five agencies listed. This high rate of usage of Social Security benefits was also reflected in patients' reports of actual receipt of payments during the year

Table 4-5.   Reported Application for and Receipt of
Benefits from Selected Sources
Base N = 205

Source of Assistance	Percent and Number of Year 8 Population Who Ever Applied	Percent and Number of Year 8 Population Reporting Receipt During Preceding Year
Social Security	26.3 (54)	
Retirement benefits		14.6 (30)
Disability benefits		10.2 (21)
Supplemental Security Income (SSI)		1.0 (2)
Veterans' benefits	25.4 (52)	15.6 (32)
Private insurance disability benefits	19.0 (39)	5.9 (12)
Worker's Compensation	12.7 (26)	1.5 (3)
Public assistance (Welfare)	4.4 (9)	2.9 (6)

prior to Year 8. Many of the men had either reached retirement age by Year 8 or been forced to leave their jobs because of their heart condition: 15% of the Year 8 population reported receipt of Social Security retirement benefits, and 10% of Social Security disability benefits, during the preceding year. Of the 54 patients who reported ever applying for any kind of Social Security benefits, 85% ($N = 46$) were currently receiving them. Our data do not permit us to report the reasons for the discrepancy between application for and current receipt of benefits, whether they be rejection of claims, improvement of health, or other causes. In several cases, at least, patients reported that they were still waiting for their applications to be processed and approved. If a patient had applied for Social Security retirement benefits, and eligibility seemed to be indicated by other information in the interview (aged 62 or over), he was classified as a retirement recipient for purposes of our statistical analysis of retirement. Using this method of classification, of all Social Security applicants in our study population, 58% were recipients or impending recipients of retirement benefits. Of total applicants, 35% were receiving disability payments, and 8% both disability and retirement benefits. Recipients of Supplemental Security Income were eliminated from the analysis, since only two men reported receiving these benefits.

Of the 46 current recipients of Social Security, over half had been receiving aid for more than 2 years, and 30% for over 5 years. Thirty-five percent ($N = 6$) of those receiving only disability benefits, 24% ($N = 6$) of those receiving only retirement benefits, and 50% ($N = 2$) of those receiving both had received payments for 5 or more years. Thus, within the population, there is a small core of men who have made continued use of Social Security resources over a period of many years.

Over two-thirds ($N = 31$) of patients receiving Social Security benefits at Year 8 characterized the payments as inadequate, which is quite understandable in view of continuing inflation. Of those patients who had received Social Security retirement benefits in the past year, one-third ($N = 10$) received less than $1,999, 62% less than $2,999. Of those men reporting receipt of Social Security disability benefits during the year before the Year 8 interview, 70% received less than $3,000.

Correlates of Use of Physician Services

Age and Use of Physician Services.   Older people characteristically make greater use of health services (Aday & Eichhorn, 1972). In our study, too, the oldest heart patients, those aged 65 to 70, reported the heaviest utilization of physicians as measured by number of doctors consulted and volume of visits. Although men aged 65 to 70 were less than 20% of the total population at Year 8, they accounted for more than half of those patients using four or more physicians. More than half the men aged 65 to 70 had seen a physician six times or more, compared to a quarter of the patients aged 40 to 49.

A U-shaped or bimodal distribution seemed to emerge when age was cross-tabulated with use of selected health services. As Table 4-6 suggests, the oldest and the youngest age groups tended to utilize these health services somewhat more heavily.

No significant differences between age groups were found with regard to types of doctors consulted or reasons for seeing a doctor. When regular checkups are examined separately, however, those in the 65 to 70 age group seem to differ significantly from the rest of the population. Only 37% of those 65 and older who consulted a doctor did so for routine checkups only, compared to 55% of men 64 and under.

Educational Level and Use of Physician Services.   Although some literature has suggested a positive relationship between educational level and use of physicians, especially for preventive services, this pattern was not borne out in the heart-patient population. We found no relationship between educational level and (1) consulting a doctor, (2) number of doctors seen, or (3) number of visits to doctors. However, education does appear to be related to maintenance of a continuous relationship with a physician. Almost three-quarters of the patients in the highest educational category had the same regular physician at Year 8 as at Year 1, compared to only a little more than half the patients with less than a high school diploma (see Table 4-7).

Occupational Level and Use of Physician Services.   Among those currently employed at Year 8, there were no statistically signifi-

Table 4-6. Patient Age at Year 8 and Selected Indices of Health Services Utilization at Year 8

Patient Age at Year 8	Total Number of Patients (N = 205)	Percent Visiting a Clinic or Emergency Room in Preceding Year	Percent Contacting One or More Health-Related Professional Services Since Year 1*	Percent Consulting Three or More Physicians in Preceding Year
40-49	27	51.9 (14)	48.1 (13)	22.2 (6)
50-54	40	40.0 (16)	32.5 (13)	12.5 (5)
55-59	50	28.0 (14)	28.0 (14)	10.0 (5)
60-64	52	34.6 (18)	34.6 (18)	19.2 (10)
65-70	36	50.0 (18)	44.4 (16)	33.3 (12)

*The professional services listed in the interview schedule appear in Table 4-3.

115

Table 4-7.   Use of Services of Same Cardiac-Care Physicians at Year 1
             and Year 8: By Educational Level, Occupational Level, Total
             Family Income at Year 8, and Number of Hospitalizations

	Total Number Who had Regular Physician for Cardiac Care at Year 8*	Percent Reporting Care by Same Physician at Both Year 1 and Year 8
Educational Level		
One Year of College or More	44	72.7 (32)
High School Graduate	47	61.7 (29)
Three Years of High School or Less	61	54.1 (33)
Chi-square = 3.76, d.f. = 2, p<.20		
Occupational Level[†]		
Professional, Managerial	25	72.0 (18)
White Collar	52	69.2 (36)
Skilled Blue Collar	19	68.4 (13)
Semiskilled and Un- skilled Blue Collar	25	48.0 (12)
Retired	31	48.4 (15)
Chi-square = 7.05, d.f. = 4, p<.20		
Total Family Income at Year 8		
$15,000 or More	74	75.7 (56)
$10,000-$14,999	42	45.2 (19)
$9,999 or Less	35	51.4 (18)
Chi-square = 12.48, d.f. = 2, p<.01		
Number of Hospitali- zations since Year 1		
None	52	67.3 (35)
1	42	66.7 (28)
2-3	39	56.4 (22)
4 or More	19	47.4 (9)
Chi-square = 3.25, d.f. = 3, NS		

*"Don't know" and non-response have been omitted.

†For discussion of occupational classifications, see Note 1, Chapter 3.

cant differences between occupational levels with regard to number of doctors seen or total volume of physician visits. Retired
patients, however, reported more utilization of physicians than
the rest of the population. For example, 18% of the retired men
($N = 51$) and only 6% of the employed population had seen

four or more doctors. Almost half the retired men (45%) reported six or more doctor visits during the preceding year, compared to 24% of the working patients. These findings might be due to the fact that retired patients were usually older men. Among employed patients, no significant differences were found between occupational levels with regard to use of either private or clinic physicians at Year 8. These findings were not modified when controlled for age.

Employed patients in the upper occupational groups were more likely to have visited their physicians only for checkups than those in the lower occupational categories. Seventy-one percent of the highest occupational group had seen a physician for a checkup only, compared with only 31% of the lowest occupational group. These findings may reflect possible real health differences, as well as different orientations to preventive care between occupational groups.

While the numbers are too small for detailed statistical analysis, we noted a greater tendency for the lower occupational groups and the retired to have changed heart-care doctors since Year 1. Only 48% of the semiskilled and unskilled and 48% of the retired men had the same coronary-care doctor at Year 8 as at Year 1, compared to 72% of those in the highest professional category (see Table 4-7).

Total Family Income and Use of Physician Services.   Although income has historically been positively associated with volume of physicians' services used, new methods of financing medical care for people with low incomes have presumably narrowed the gap (Andersen, Lion, & Anderson, 1976). Total family income at Year 8 was not related to either number of doctors seen or total number of physician visits. However, there was a tendency for middle and lower income patients to use more clinic doctors, and for those with higher family incomes to use more private physicians. These figures support the conclusion that people with low incomes more often seek physicians' services at clinics or emergency rooms.

Of patients who had seen a doctor in the year prior to the Year 8 interview, those in the highest income category were most likely to have visited the physician for a routine checkup only. Sixty-one percent ($N = 52$) of those who reported total family incomes of $15,000 or more did so, compared to 49% (N = 22) of those with family incomes of $9,999 or less. Whether the patient had the same regular doctor at Year 8 as he had at Year 1 was significantly positively related to total family income. Of those men with regular doctors at Year 8, 51% of those with total family incomes of $9,999 or less had the same doctor, compared with 76% of those with incomes of $15,000 or more.

Social Security and Worker's Compensation: Correlates of Use of Services

Social Security. Some of the factors associated with Social Security usage at Year 8 were: age, educational level, retirement status, total family income, and hospitalization experience. As expected, the oldest men were most likely to have applied for Social Security and to have received benefits of various types during the year prior to Year 8 (see Table 4-8).Of the 22 patients who reported receiving disability payments in the past year, 64% (N = 14) had less than a high school diploma (see Table 4-9). However, there were no significant differences among occupational levels of employed men with regard to application for or receipt of Social Security benefits.

Of the retired men, 78% (N = 40) had at some time applied for Social Security, including retirement and disability benefits. A fifth (N = 10) of the retired men, however, reported that they had never applied for Social Security. For the most part, these patients were former federal or municipal employees who had retired early, were collecting comfortable pensions, and were still too young to qualify for Social Security retirement benefits.

Among the 40 retired men who were receiving Social Security payments at Year 8, 27 were receiving retirement benefits only, 10 disability benefits only, and 3 both disability and retirement benefits. Thus over one-quarter (N = 13) of all retired men in the Year 8 population were receiving Social Security disability benefits. Those receiving only disability payments were usually below the minimum age for receipt of retirement benefits. All attributed their disability to their heart conditions.

A strong negative relationship between total family income and application for Social Security benefits was found at Year 8.

Table 4-8. Patient Application for Social Security Benefits at Any Time and
Types of Benefits Received During Previous 12 Months. By Age.

Age at Year 8

| | *Application for Social Security Benefits* | | |
	Yes *Percent (N)*	*No* *Percent (N)*	*Number of* *Patients*
40-49	18.5 (5)	81.5 (22)	27
50-59	5.6 (5)	94.4 (85)	90
60-70	50.6 (44)	49.4 (43)	87
Total	54	150	204*

Chi-square = 47.08, d.f. = 2, p<.001

| | *Receipt of Social Security Benefits by Type* | | | |
	Retirement *Only*	*Disability* *Only*	*Retirement* *and Disability*	*Number of* *Patients*
40-49	0	(3)	0	3
50-59	0	(5)	0	5
60-70	68.2 (30)	22.7 (10)	9.1 (4)	44
Total	30	18	4	52†

*"Don't know" responses have been eliminated.

†Two men who had applied for Social Security benefits but did not report receipt of payments have been omitted. These men were not imminent retirees, and the reasons for nonreceipt of benefits are unknown.

This association was attributable only in part to the fact that retirees were most likely to have applied for benefits, and tended to be in the lower income categories (see Table 4-10).

The most frequently hospitalized patients were most likely to have utilized Social Security resources of one type or another. Sixty-eight percent of patients with four or more hospitalizations had applied for Social Security, compared with only 16% of those not hospitalized. Two-thirds of the 22 patients with four or more hospitalizations reported receipt of Social Security disability benefits, compared with 16% of those with no hospitalizations (see

Table 4-9.   Patient Application for Social Security Benefits at Any
             Time and Types of Benefits Received During Previous 12
             Months. By Educational Level.

Educational Level

| | Application for Social Security Benefits | | |
	Yes Percent (N)	No Percent (N)	Number of Patients
One Year of College or More	18.6 (11)	81.4 (48)	59
High School Graduate	19.4 (12)	80.6 (50)	62
3 Years of High School or Less	37.3 (31)	62.7 (52)	83
Total	54	150	204[*]

Chi-square = 8.52, d.f. = 2, p<.05

| | Receipt of Social Security Benefits by Type | | | |
	Retire- ment Only	Disability Only	Retirement and Disability	Number of Patients
One Year of College or More	63.6 (7)	27.3 (3)	9.1 (1)	11
High School Graduate	63.6 (7)	27.3 (3)	9.1 (1)	11
3 Years of High School or Less	53.3 (16)	40.0 (12)	6.7 (2)	30
Total	30	18	4	52[†]

[*]"Don't know" responses have been eliminated.

[†]Two men who had applied for Social Security benefits but did not report receipt of payments have been omitted. These men were not imminent retirees, and the reasons for nonreceipt of benefits are unknown.

Table 4-11). In general, then, the patients most in need of Social Security benefits were indeed seeking and receiving them.

Worker's Compensation as a Resource.   The less educated were more likely ever to have applied for Worker's Compensation: 18% of the patients with less than a high school diploma had done

Table 4-10.   Patient Application for Social Security Benefits at Any Time.
By Total Family Income at Year 8.

| Total Family Income at Year 8 | Application for Social Security Benefits | | |
	Yes Percent (N)	No Percent (N)	Number of Patients (N = 205)*
Total Year 8 Population			
$9,999 or less	55.8 (29)	44.2 (23)	52
$10,000 - $14,999	26.3 (15)	73.7 (42)	57
$15,000 or more	9.6 (9)	90.4 (85)	94
Total	53	150	203
	Chi-square = 37.04, d.f. = 2, p<.001		
Employed Men Only			
$9,999 or less	27.3 (6)	72.7 (16)	22
$10,000 - $14,999	2.7 (1)	97.3 (36)	37
$15,000 or more	2.4 (2)	97.6 (80)	82
Total	9	132	141[†]
Retired Men Only			
$9,999 or less	91.7 (22)	8.3 (2)	24
$10,000 - $14,999	80.0 (12)	20.0 (3)	15
$15,000 or more	54.5 (6)	45.5 (5)	11
Total	40	10[‡]	50

*"Don't know" responses have been omitted.   Information was not avail-
able on one patient's total family income.

[†]Men unemployed but not retired at Year 8 have been omitted.

[‡]Men in this category had been in occupations in which they were not
covered by Social Security.

so, compared with only 3% of those with some college education.
It is likely that more highly educated patients are better able to
continue employment in their work settings and are also able to
modify the requirements of the job, and that the college educated
have other pension plans and savings.

    In general, the patients most likely to seek Worker's Com-

Table 4-11. Patient Application for Social Security Benefits at Any Time
            and Types of Benefits Received During Previous 12 Months.
            By Number of Patient Hospitalizations From Year 1 to Year 8.

*Number of Hospitalizations
from Year 1 to Year 8*

	Application for Social Security Benefits		
	Yes *Percent (N)*	*No* *Percent (N)*	*Number of* *Patients*
None	16.0 (12)	84.0 (63)	75
1	20.4 (11)	79.6 (43)	54
2-3	30.2 (16)	69.8 (37)	53
4 or more	68.2 (15)	31.8 (7)	22
Total	54	150	204*

Chi-square = 25.29, d.f. = 3, p<.005

	Receipt of Social Security Benefits by Type			
	Retirement *Only*	*Disability* *Only*	*Retirement* *and Disability*	*Number of* *Patients*
None	81.8 (9)	18.2 (2)	-- --	11
1	54.5 (6)	27.3 (3)	18.2 (2)	11
2-3	66.7 (10)	33.3 (5)	-- --	15
4 or more	33.3 (5)	53.4 (8)	13.3 (2)	15
Total	30	18	4	52†

*"Don't know" responses have been eliminated.

†Two men who had applied for Social Security benefits but did not report receipt of payments have been omitted. These men were not imminent retirees, and the reasons for nonreceipt of benefits are unknown.

pensation tended to be the oldest, in the lowest income, occupational, and educational categories, and to report the highest numbers of hospitalizations. These patients appeared to show a greater proclivity to claim disability, perhaps because they were unable to redefine their jobs and had no other financial resources on which to draw. As is well known, older persons also have more difficulty getting new jobs.

SUMMARY

Eight years after their first myocardial infarction the heart patients continue to manifest the high rate of utilization of physicians' services documented at Year 1. Patients' reports suggest relatively frequent and regular interaction with their doctors, continuity of care, and apparent satisfaction with physician services.

As we might expect, the oldest patients tended to report more use of physician services. A positive relationship was found between social status and utilization of private physicians, and a corresponding negative association emerged between socioeconomic status and use of clinic doctors.

Patients in the highest educational, occupational, and family income categories, and those with the fewest hospitalizations, were most likely to have the same regular heart doctor at Year 8 as Year 1. Conversely, those with the least education, lowest occupational levels and total family incomes, and most hospitalizations were most likely to have changed doctors.

Educational groups in this population did not differ significantly with regard to physician utilization. However, patients in the highest income and occupational groups did report in greater proportions than other men that their only reason for seeing a doctor was for a routine checkup. This difference might reflect real health differences as well as attitudes toward preventive care.

The study population as a whole made substantial use of clinics, emergency rooms, and hospitals. However, utilization of other health professionals and agencies was minimal, with the exception of some sources of predominantly financial assistance, notably Social Security. This finding is particularly striking given the proliferation of professionals and agencies in the Boston area and the variety of illness-related problems in a considerable segment of the heart patient study group over the years.

The patients most likely to report utilization of Social Security resources tended to be retired, in the oldest age group, in the lowest educational and income categories, and to report the most hospitalizations. Application for Worker's Compensation benefits was also negatively related to education, age, total family income, and occupational level, and positively associated with hospitalization experience.

NOTE

1. This apparent concentration of recent hospitalizations may be partially accounted for by a tendency to forget such events greater than 1 year distant. For a review of this problem, see Jenkins, Hurst, & Rose, 1979.

Chapter 5

PHYSICIANS AND PATIENTS

Advice and Compliance Orientation

INTRODUCTION

Within the "armory of resources" available to the patients in this study, the physician is clearly among the most central. As we have seen in Chapter 4, physicians are a far more prominent source of guidance and support than other professionals, hospitals, or social service agencies. Most patients reported regular interaction with their doctors and continuity of care, and they presented a general picture of relative satisfaction with physician services.

Eight years after their first heart attacks, as we have seen, the current physical status and health histories of the men varied considerably. However, regardless of their current level of health or degree of disability and impairment, the patients shared a major characteristic: all had chronic illness in the form of arteriosclerotic heart disease. Their cardiac status would inevitably be a factor in medical management for the rest of their lives.

In fact, over 90% of the patients reported at Year 8 that they were currently under the supervision or care of a physician and that they had been given instructions and advice as part of the medical regimen. While some had immediate health problems other than heart disease, the population as a whole shared a common core of medical instructions.

Thus, for nearly all the respondents, the medical regimen was an important element in the doctor-patient relationship. In the social contract between the two participants, it was assumed that for his own benefit the patient would take heed of the physician's advice and adhere to it. This chapter examines some aspects of that compliance, reviewing it in terms of data from the 8-year follow-up period. Our principal focus is upon two aspects: (1) "compliance orientation"—or proclivity to comply; and (2) reported compliance behavior, using cigarette smoking as a case in point.

That compliance with physician advice is of critical importance in the care of heart patients is a widely accepted precept in medicine. In recent years it has received an increasing amount of attention and analysis. The professional literature ranges from hortatory accounts and philosophical statements to empirical studies of compliance with medical regimens and with health education efforts (see, for example, Becker et al., 1972, 1974; Johannsen et al., 1966; Marston, 1970; Mitchell, 1974). Various theoretical models have been developed to help explain and predict compliance behavior, in regard both to specific illnesses and to illness in general (Hochbaum, 1958; Kasl & Cobb, 1966; Kegeles, 1963, 1969; Kirscht, 1974; Rosenstock, 1960). Numerous efforts are underway to improve measures of compliance through the use of standardized observations, including blood tests, urinalysis, physical measurement, and systematic reporting of patient behavior by research personnel.

The problems of studying and measuring compliance are relatively well known and need no detailed recapitulation here. Some few examples perhaps can suffice. Unfortunately, there are few valid instruments available for measuring conformity with advice which involves complex behavior, which must be carried out for a long period, and which is not easily amenable to scrutiny. It is hard to classify levels of actual compliance, particularly when dealing with areas of advice which are varied and of differing levels of specificity.[1] Further one cannot assume that compliance in one area is indicative of compliance in others; this matter is an empirical question on which adequate research has yet to be done. The use of "objective" measures of compliance is also accompanied by problems of its own, including patient dissembling and temporary alterations of behavior, intrusions on privacy, and cost (Gordis, 1976).

In brief, as we pointed out in our earlier report (Croog & Levine, 1977), compliance behavior is an area in which major conceptual and methodological advances still remain to be made. Our approach here, therefore, is to proceed conservatively in reporting and interpreting our findings.

COMPLIANCE BEHAVIOR AND COMPLIANCE ORIENTATION: SOME KEY DISTINCTIONS

In an article some years ago, Davis usefully pointed out that "compliance behavior" should be kept conceptually separate from "compliant attitudes." As an attitude, he wrote, compliance consists of a willingness or orientation toward doing what the doctor advises. "In its behavioral aspect, however, compliance can be said to exist only when the patient actually carries out his doctor's orders" (Davis, 1968).

Our concern is with one key dimension of the compliance phenomenon: "compliance orientation." This is operationally defined as the degree of expressed willingness of the patient to comply with an item of advice, as indicated by his report of past and/or intended compliance behavior. For our analytic purposes we view the responses as reflecting a compliance attitude or frame of mind—a willingness or intention to obey the instructions of the physician.

In interviews at Year 8, patients were given a list of areas on which physicians commonly give advice to persons with heart disease. The list included such areas as medications, diet, exercise, smoking, and the like. The men were asked to specify the items on which they had received advice. For each of these, they were then asked, "How well have you been able to follow the doctor's advice?" Responses were coded: "completely," "for the most part," "somewhat," or "not at all."

The data were reclassified in terms of three categories for analysis: complete compliance, partial compliance, and noncompliance. The two intermediate response groups, "for the most part" and "somewhat" were treated as partial compliance. The same format and procedure was followed also at Week 7 and Year 1 in our earlier study, permitting comparative analysis on essentially the same items over time.

For some analytic purposes we further combined partial compliance and noncompliance into a single category, indicating an orientation other than complete compliance. We have used two terms to distinguish the types of compliance orientation in a brief fashion: (1) positive complier and (2) noncomplier. The positive complier is the patient who reports complete compliance with the advice. The noncomplier refers here to the patient who is characterized by complete or partial noncompliance.

Our inclusion of "partial compliance" in the noncompliance orientation category is based upon the rationale that reported partial compliance is more indicative of noncompliance than of actual compliance. From the medical standpoint, partial compliers often may be as problematic as noncompliers. Clearly, patients who are given medications for treatment of their heart disease but only partially comply belong in another category than patients who cooperate fully in taking their medicine.

Our focus on compliance orientation is, of course, quite different from a focus on actual patient behavior with regard to physicians' advice. It is basically concerned, however, with one of the primary and essential elements in most compliance behavior relating to the medical regimen—a favorable orientation toward following through with the instructions and guidance. As research by others has shown, a positive compliance orientation is more strongly associated with actual compliance than is an ambivalent or negative intention.[2] Our use of the notion of compliance orientation also permits a review of patient responses to differing types of advice, varying in content, degree of specificity, ease of fulfillment, and emotional overtone. At a later point in the chapter, as we have indicated, we will consider one aspect of reported compliance behavior in regard to a major item in the usual medical regimen for heart patients—smoking reduction.

Medical Advice and Compliance Orientation

Patterns of Compliance Orientation: Individual Advice Items

Table 5–1 presents data on compliance orientation with regard to 10 principal areas of medical advice at Year 8. As may be seen in the third section there were only a few areas for which a majority of patients reported having received advice from their physicians (medication, weight control, diet, and smoking). We must emphasize, of course, that the table reflects only patients' perceptions and reports of advice. Obviously, the data are influenced by many factors, including patients' health status, life style, physician judgments, patient recall, and the adequacy of communication between physician and patient. However, whatever the background of influences, the reported perceptions themselves are part of the mental frame of the patients and as such may be important factors in their compliance.

On 6 of the 10 items, 50% or more of the patients reporting the advice at Year 8 can be classified as "positive compliers." These include: work, rest, exercise, alcohol consumption, medications, and sexual activity. Aside from medications, however, only a little more than half of the patients are positive compliers even in these areas. On the other four items (smoking, diet, weight control, and avoidance of quarrels), less than half of the patients indicate they are positive compliers.

In the area in which compliance orientation is strongest—medications—a specific, limited set of actions is required. Since self-medication usually requires repeated and consistent behavior, compliance can be routinized. Further, unlike most of the other advice areas, the potential health benefits of medication—and the risks of dangers of noncompliance—can more readily be perceived and understood by patients.

The percentage of men who effectively follow medical advice in each category is probably somewhat less than their reports of "positive compliance" would indicate. For example, reduction of alcohol intake may have a variety of meanings, depending on initial intake: the heavy drinker who becomes a moderate drinker is still classified as a "positive complier," along with the patient who initially drank only rarely and stops completely. Other advice from the physician, such as "get more rest"

Table 5-1. Positive Compliance Orientation Toward Physician Advice
Over Time

Item of Advice	Week 7 (N = 345)		Year 1 (N = 293)		Year 8 (N = 205)	
	Percent Reporting Receipt of Advice	Of Those Advised, Percent With Positive Compliance Orientation	Percent Reporting Receipt of Advice	Of Those Advised, Percent With Positive Compliance Orientation	Percent Reporting Receipt of Advice	Of Those Advised, Percent With Positive Compliance Orientation
Medications	89.0	88.3	66.3	90.2	50.7	88.5
Diet	80.0	63.4	65.0	48.8	56.1	34.8
Smoking	73.0	58.7	65.0	44.2	58.5	41.7
Work	71.3	79.7	64.6	59.2	42.4	55.2
Weight control	65.5	54.4	74.1	42.3	67.8	29.5
Resting	54.2	64.2	49.5	55.2	32.7	52.2
Alcohol consumption	50.4	78.7	36.6	63.5	32.2	62.1
Avoiding quarrels	42.9	42.6	40.4	22.8	19.5	37.5
Exercise	39.1	75.6	74.1	51.6	48.8	49.0
Sexual activity	3.2*	—	18.2	56.6	9.8	60.0

*Information on this item is based on responses to an open-end question at Week 7 concerning additional areas of physician advice. Patients were not questioned at Week 7 regarding compliance with advice on sexual activity.

and "exercise more," is sufficiently diffuse, so that a broad range of behavior can be defined as compliant.

Hence, these data on compliance orientation serve also to point up a potentially substantial degree of nonconformity with medical advice in actual health care behavior. We can raise questions about real conformity among those who say they comply. And as we have noted, we can assume strongly that those without a positive compliance orientation are less likely to follow medical advice than those with a positive orientation.

Whether or not the compliance with medical advice in each area is rational or therapeutic is not our concern here. Although there are strong positive indications, the precise efficacy and benefit of all the items of advice have not yet been established definitively. There is still controversy on each, as reflected in the scientific and popular literature (Kannel & Dawber, 1972; Mann, 1977). In providing the advice, the patients' physicians have obviously made medical judgments as to the desirability and benefit of compliance. And in various ways, the patients have made their own judgments, as seen in their reported action or noncompliance. Unfortunately we do not have the multi-dimensional data which would permit exploration of the complex issues concerning the relationship of compliance to long-term health outcome.

Because of the longitudinal, prospective design of this research, we can examine patterns of reported physician advice and compliance as they appeared 7 and 8 years earlier—in the first year following the initial myocardial infarction. These materials are drawn from interviews at Week 7 and at Year 1; they appear in sections 1 and 2 of Table 5–1.

Physician Advice Over Time.   A comparison of findings on reported advice at Week 7, Year 1, and Year 8 readily shows long-term changes in the experience of the patient population. On the whole, higher proportions of each cohort reported receipt of advice on most items at Week 7 and Year 1, those times closest to the first, acute phases of the illness. The percentages reporting advice at Year 8 are smaller for most items. While 90% reported prescription of medications at Week 7 shortly after the acute phase, it is readily understandable that 8 years later a much smaller proportion would require medicines. At Year 8, more of the men were engaged in their usual lives, and the nature of the illness and recovery is such that fewer may have actually needed certain kinds of advice. Further, the patient and his doctor may have developed an understanding over time which rendered the repetition of particular advice unnecessary. Finally, a selective process may have been at work; many of those men most seriously ill at Week 7 and Year 1 had died by Year 8 (see Chapter 2).

Compliance Orientation Over Time.   In general, among patients receiving advice, the Year 8 pattern of compliance orientation resembles that of Year 1. At Week 7, however, during the early phase of the illness higher proportions of patients reported positive compliance orientation on nine items than at Year 1 or Year 8. The sole exception is in the case of medications. Here 90% of the patients in each cohort reported positive compliance at all three stages.

Although the elements which underlie positive compliance are complex, these data suggest differences in the level of concern or anxiety about the illness over time. Initially, at Week 7, the patients may be responding with promised conformity to advice and obedience to authority, employing this as one mechanism of coping with the new experience of a life-threatening illness. Over the longer term, however, a more flexible attitude toward the physician's advice may develop. It should be noted, parenthetically, that although the positive compliance rates were higher at Week 7 than at Year 1 or Year 8, considerable proportions of the patients manifested noncompliant orientations even in the early period after the first heart attack.

Correlates of Compliance Orientation: Year 8 and Comparisons with Previous Stages.   We have examined our data on compliance orientation in relation to two principal sets of possible correlates: (1) current variables associated with compliance orientation as of the time of the Year 8 interview and (2) antecedent variables based on information from the base-line study 7 years earlier.

The variables we selected for analysis in relation to compliance orientation at Year 8 included: (1) social and personal characteristics, such as age, occupation, educational level; (2) self-rated psychological characteristics; (3) current health status, as indicated by such measures, as self-reported symptoms, visits to physicians, and physician ratings; (4) hospitalization history; (5) record of previous reported compliance orientation; and (6) patient conceptions of factors in the etiology of the illness. (A listing of these variables and ways in which they were coded appears in Note 4.)

Our analysis was guided by hypotheses suggested by previous studies as well as by our own tentative assumptions about potentially relevant correlates. Some of these were that level of reported compliance orientation varies: (1) by social status level, as indicated by educational level and by occupational type; (2) by age; and (3) by personality characteristics. We also hypothesized that: (4) those men most severely ill were likely to report higher compliance orientation than those who were least ill; and (5) that previous compliance orientation is a useful predictor of current compliance orientation. These examples are based on findings reported in such reviews as those by Becker and Maiman (1975), Davis and Eichhorn (1963), Marston (1970), Kasl (1975), and Sackett and Haynes (1976).

Compliance orientation with regard to each of eight physician advice items (work, rest, exercise, smoking, alcohol, diet, weight, and medications) was crosstabulated against the individual independent variables. The item, medications, could be examined only in a limited way because nearly 90% of the patients were reported compliers and the number of noncompliers was insufficient for most analyses. The analysis produced relatively few statistically significant associations. As some of these findings could have occurred by chance, special caution must be exercised in interpretation.

Although some investigators have found educational and occupational level useful in studying compliance, these variables were not associated with compliance orientation on the individual items we examined. Nor were the psychological self-rating items related in any consistent pattern with the compliance orientation measures. Two exceptions appeared. Those who described themselves as "easily depressed" were less likely to report positive compliance orientation on "avoiding quarrels," and advice on "rest." Men who characterized themselves as "in a hurry" were significantly less likely to comply with advice on work.

Patients' perceptions about the etiology of their heart attacks were not associated with adherence to physician advice. For example, men who believed that "diet" or "being overweight" was an important factor in the development of their illness were not more inclined to comply with advice on these matters than men who did not hold such beliefs. Whether or not men believed smoking to be a contributing factor in their heart disease was not related to their reported compliance with advice on smoking. Clearly, the degree to which knowledge or beliefs are reflected in behavior is limited (see also Croog & Richards, 1977).

Measures of current health status also were not associated with compliance orientation on the individual advice items. These measures included recent symptoms reported, physician ratings of functional capacity, recency of visits to a physician, and hospitalization for heart disease during the 2 years prior to the Year 8 interview.

Correlates of Compliance Orientations at Three Time Points: Week 7, Year 1, Year 8. These findings at Year 8 are consistent with those which we obtained in our earlier study of the first year after the heart attack (1977). We reported that at Week 7 and Year 1 the level of compliance orientation was generally unrelated to social and personal characteristics, psychological self-rating items, number of symptoms reported, total number of items of advice received, and patient rehospitalization during the year. Thus, for the most part, patterns evident early in the illness continued to be manifest in our follow-up study years later.

However, two sets of variables—age and prior compliance orientation—deserve note here because of consistent association with particular compliance orientation items. Older men reported significantly higher positive compliance orientation at Year 8 on a series of advice items. The respective gamma measures of association between *age* and compliance orientation on the advice items were: alcohol consumption (.56), weight control (.34), dietary practices (.44), and use of medications (.48). It should be noted that our results are not generally consistent with findings of several other studies with somewhat different populations and methodologies. In most of these other studies, age was not associated with compliance (Cuskey et al., 1971; Rae, 1972; Weintraub et al., 1973).

Prior compliance orientation at Year 1 on a number of advice items was also related to compliance orientation at Year 8 on analogous items. When compliance orientations reported at Years 1 and 8 were compared for selected items of advice, the following gamma associations were found: smoking, .85; exercise, .50; weight control, .55; and diet, .45.

Ninety percent of patients who were positive compliers on medications at Year 1 remained so at Year 8. However, most of the few earlier noncompliers changed to a more positive compliance orientation 7 years later. Thus, a pattern of high compliance was maintained and noncompliance appeared to have been modified over time with regard to medications.

High consistency was also found between positive compliance orientations reported at Week 7 and at Year 8 in regard to two items: advice on smoking and diet. Thus, patients who indicated at Week 7 that they were following their physicians' advice on smoking and diet were likely to report positive compliance orientation on these items 8 years later.

These findings present suggestive evidence about the persistence of particular positive attitudinal orientations over extended periods of time.

The Compliance Orientation Index

We now turn from consideration of individual items of physician advice to appraisal of patient response to the total series of advice items which they received. As we have seen, most patients were provided with instructions and guidance by their physicians on a number of items. However, patients vary widely in their degree of interest, ability, and motivation to comply with each item of advice. When patients receive multiple items of advice, we can differentiate between them as adhering to "none," "some," or "all" of the items of the medical regimen.

Our first inquiry centers on the pattern of patient compliance orientation toward multiple items of advice. A second issue concerns the relationship between number of items of advice received and the orientation to compliance. It is often assumed that the number of areas of advice is related to ability of the patient to respond, that "information overload" leads to poor response. Our data on a series of 10 advice items permit some examination of this question.

A third issue concerns the variables which may be associated with the total pattern of compliance orientation. Do "low," "medium," and "high" compliers on multiple items differ in social and psychological characteristics? Are there useful "predictor" variables which can identify patients in terms of their probable compliance orientation?

We shall examine these three issues using the model which we employed in our earlier study in order to maximize comparability over time. In doing so, we are thus able to consider a fourth issue—the long-term stability of the compliance orientation pattern and its correlates covering a period of 8 years.

In order to examine compliance orientation as a pattern of response to a series of items, we have employed an index based on the 10 items listed in Table 5–1. The Compliance Orientation Index (or C-O Index) was calculated according to the following formula:

$$\frac{B \times 100}{A} = \text{compliance orientation percentage}$$

where A = number of items of advice reported by the patients

and B = number of items of complete compliance reported by the patient.

The results are expressed as a series of percentages for our purposes here, but we must emphasize that these computations use a small numerical base. The materials cannot be generalized, of course, beyond the analysis of this study population.

The Index serves as a means of differentiating patients, so that they can be classified in three principal categories: high, medium, and low. The data can also be arrayed as a percentage distribution for informational and comparative purposes over time. In addition, we must note that in classifying compliance orientation, we follow the same rationale as in the previous section of this chapter, using the statement of "complete compliance" as the prime criterion. Noncompliance and partial compliance are regarded as "other than complete compliance."

C-O Scores in Longitudinal Perspective.   We consider first the total pattern of compliance orientation as reported at Year 8 (see Table 5–2). Of the 185 surviving patients who were under a medical regimen at Year 8, nearly 30% indicated relatively low positive compliance. They reported "complete compliance" on only 20% or fewer of the items on which they had been advised. At the other extreme, approximately 20% manifested "high com-

Table 5-2.   Compliance Orientation Index Scores.
Cohorts at Week 7, Year 1 and Year 8

| | Frequency Distribution of Patients | | | | | |
| | Week 7 | | Year 1 | | Year 8 | |
Compliance Orientation Index Score[*]	N	Percent	N	Percent	N	Percent
0-9	6	1.7	31	11.0	43	23.2
10-19	11	3.2	13	4.6	9	4.9
20-29	11	3.2	31	11.0	19	10.3
30-39	14	4.1	27	9.5	17	9.2
40-49	11	3.2	21	7.4	12	6.5
50-59	45	13.1	46	16.3	20	10.8
60-69	42	12.2	27	9.5	21	11.3
70-79	59	17.2	25	8.8	9	4.9
80-89	69	20.0	28	9.9	11	5.9
90-99	5	1.5	0	0	0	0
100	71	20.6	34	12.0	24	13.0
Total[†]	344	100.0	283	100.0	185	100.0
Mean Compliance Orientation Index Score	71.3		52.8		45.6	
Standard Deviation	24.1		29.4		32.5	

[*]Score represents the percent of items of advice received to which the patient has indicated positive compliance orientation. See text.

[†]Men who reported receiving no advice from their physicians have been excluded from the total.

pliance", reporting positive compliance on 80% or more of the advice items. Perhaps most striking is the fact that over half the men on a medical regimen (54%) had Index scores of less than 50%. In other words, over half were less than strong compliers on most of the physician advice items in their medical regimen.

Some perspectives on distributions at Year 8 are provided by the data on C-O Index scores for the cohorts at Week 7 and Year 1 (Table 5–2). The mean Compliance Index score at Week 7 was the highest, and the mean scores for the subsequent time points were substantially lower. Thus, reported compliance with the medical regimen was greatest in the initial period after the first heart attack. It was least at 8 years among those men who were still supposed to be following a regimen of medical advice.

In the Week 7 cohort, relatively few men (5%) had C-O scores of less than 20%. At Year 1, 15% of the men were in that lowest category, and at Year 8, nearly 30% of the men had scores of under 20%. A similar pattern is evident at the upper end of the scale; in contrast to Year 1 and Year 8, over 40% of the respondents at Week 7 had C-O scores of 80% or more.

The data thus far concerned cohorts at three time points, but they do not indicate changes by individuals over time. To explore the matter more adequately, we examined a select group of patients, those who participated in the study at all three time points and who reported receiving advice from their physicians ($N = 181$). When we trace these same individuals over the 8 years, a pattern of reduction in compliance emerges, which is consistent with the cohort data.

Thus, in this core population over time there was a reduction in the percentage reporting the highest compliance orientation scores. For example, at Week 7, 42% of these men had C-O Index scores of 80 to 100, whereas at Year 8 only 19% of this same group had scores in this range. Similarly, at the other extreme, 30% had C-O Index scores of 60 or lower at Week 7, but at Year 8, 65% of this core population was in this category of least reported compliance.

Information Overload and C-O Scores.   Is compliance orientation in this population related to the number of items of advice provided by the physician? We pursued the issue of information overload in the medical regimen by examining the number of advice items in relation to the patients' C-O scores. No statistically significant association was found.

Our results are influenced in part, of course, by the number of advice items. If physicians advised one set of patients on 250 matters and another set of men on 1 or 2 matters, it is obvious that the potential for complete compliance would be greater in the latter group. However, we have limited the list to 10 principal items on which advice is commonly provided in clinical cardiac care. In this context, therefore, the finding seems clear. It is also noteworthy that in our earlier study similar findings of lack of association emerged at Week 7 and Year 1, on these variables.

The Compliance Orientation Score and Its Correlates. Are there particular variables of a social, psychological, or demographic nature which can help account for Compliance Index scores? Are there correlates of the Compliance Index scores which might also serve as predictors of subsequent scores on the Index?

To pursue these questions, we divided the total population receiving advice at Year 8 into approximate terciles on the basis of C-O Index scores. The three subsegments of the study group can be characterized simply as "high," "medium," and "low" compliers.

Compliance Orientation Index Score at Year 8	N	Percent
High: 60–100	65	35.1
Medium: 20–59	68	36.8
Low: 0–19	52	28.1
	185[3]	100.0

As in the case of individual physician advice items, a series of crosstabulations were carried out using the three-category C-O Index scores. The independent variables we examined included age, education, occupational level, selected psychological self-rating items, and measures of health. (See Note 4 for listing.)

Among these possible correlates, the only one which showed meaningful association with C-O score was age. This finding is consistent with the outcome of our earlier analysis of individual items. As Table 5–3 shows, the greater the age, the higher the proportion of men indicating compliance.

The finding on age and reported compliance orientation is difficult to compare with other studies because of differences in methods, study populations, and the illnesses of the respondents. In general, conflicting evidence appears. For example, in a review of the literature on compliance, Davis (1966) reported that older men in the age group 46 to 65 were poorer compliers with medical advice than younger men. Most research has revealed no consistent evidence of a relationship between age and compliance (Becker et al., 1972; Marston, 1970; Sackett & Haynes, 1976).

Our finding of an association between age and compliance orientation is not attributable to poorer health among the older men. In the first place, as we have seen in Chapter 2, age was not related to our measures of health and functional capacity. To pursue this empirical observation further, we carried out a number of statistical tests. We used two measures of illness: (1) record of rehospitalization and (2) report of current symptoms. Con-

Table 5-3. Compliance Orientation Index Scores at Year 8 by Patient Age[*]

| Age at Week 7 | Compliance Orientation Index Score at Year 8 in Terciles[†] | | | | | | Total |
| | High | | Medium | | Low | | |
	N	Percent	N	Percent	N	Percent	N
30–39	3	15.8	5	26.3	11	57.9	19
40–44	5	21.7	10	43.5	8	34.8	23
45–49	14	30.4	18	39.1	14	30.4	46
50–54	22	44.0	17	34.0	11	22.0	50
55–60	21	44.7	18	38.3	8	17.0	47
Total N	65		68		52		185[‡]

[*]Chi-square = 16.04, d.f. = 8, $p<.05$, gamma = .30.

[†]High: 60-100; Medium: 20-59; Low: 0-19.

[‡]Twenty men who reported receiving no advice from their physicians have been excluded from the table.

trolling for level of illness, the same positive association appeared between age and C-O score at Year 8.

Another variable which predicted compliance at Year 8 was previous score on the C-O Index 7 and 8 years earlier. In a separate analysis we compared the C-O score at Week 7, Year 1, and Year 8. The core study population selected was the group at Year 8 who received advice from their physicians ($N = 185$).

The results showed a significant association between C-O scores from Week 7 to Year 1 for this surviving group (Gamma = .48, chi-square = 20.32, d.f. = 4, $p < .001$. Further there was an association between the Year 1 score and the C-O score at Year 8, although the relationship was somewhat weaker (Gamma = .25, chi-square = 10.60, d.f. = 4, $p < .05$). However, no significant relationship was found between the Week 7 and Year 8 scores.

What do these data tell us? There appears to be a pattern of continuity in reported compliance from one time point to another, although its strength declines over the years. We have no information, of course, on the periods between time points. But the data do suggest once again that previous compliance orientation may be one of the most useful predictors of subsequent compliance orientation. It has long been an operating principle in studies of task performance that past behavior is one of the best predictors of future behavior, and our findings on persistence of compliance orientation over time seem to underline this point.

These results are also consistent with those which emerged in our earlier study of the year following the first heart attack. We noted a singular lack of significant associations between compliance orientation in the first year and many of the same independent variables examined here. The primary exception was the finding of a positive relationship between age and compliance orientation.

The fact that so few variables were related to compliance orientation may be a product of the types of measures used, their relative sensitivity, or their validity. Since a large number of crosstabulations were run, some of the few significant results could have emerged purely through chance. At the same time, we must also point out that our findings of few correlates of compliance orientation are congruent with a large volume of other research reports on compliance *behavior* in illness (Becker, 1979; Dunbar & Stunkard, 1979). On the whole, the continuing problems of developing reliable generalizations concerning social and psychological variables and the compliance phenomenon, may be useful in pointing toward more subtle variables and complex underlying processes in the recovery and rehabilitation of heart patients.

Thus far we have focused on reported orientation to compliance, rather than on behavior. We now turn to consideration of long-term adherence to physician instructions on a key advice item: smoking.

COMPLIANCE BEHAVIOR: AN EIGHT-YEAR PERSPECTIVE ON SMOKING[5]

Smoking is one of the most common topics on which physicians advise heart patients. Physicians' exhortations to "reduce smoking" or "give up smoking" are reinforced in the United States by newspaper and magazine articles, television announcements, the Surgeon General's Report on Smoking, programs of the American Heart Association and the American Cancer Society, and folklore concerning smoking and heart disease. Concurrent with these numerous and pervasive efforts, the proportion of smokers has declined in the past two decades in the United States. At the time of the first Surgeon General's *Report* in 1964, slightly over half the adult men in the United States were smokers; by 1975 the figure had declined to 39% (USDHEW, 1979a).

But a substantial proportion of the population continues to smoke. Antismoking health education programs have had only mixed and often minimal success (Thompson, 1978). Their record is consistent in many respects with that of other prevention-oriented programs, such as efforts in dental caries reduction, weight control, and influenza innoculation. "Success" in altering smoking behavior by individual change agents, such as physicians and therapists in modification programs, has thus far been reported primarily for limited periods, rarely exceeding a year (USDHEW, 1979b). The optimum methods of inducing populations to reduce or give up smoking are still to be identified, and theories and programs on this issue continue to proliferate.

In the case of our study population, it has been possible to appraise reported smoking behavior over a period of 8 years in a group well familiar with an illness to which smoking may predispose—heart disease. Our longitudinal approach permits examination of (1) change and stability of smoking by the heart patients; and (2) possible correlates or influences upon reported smoking behavior.

At Week 7, patients were asked a series of questions concerning their use of cigarettes, pipes, and cigars in the period previous to the heart attack. At Week 7—and subsequently at Year 1 and Year 8—they were asked about current smoking behavior. For purposes of examining change and stability, we shall here concern ourselves with cigarette smoking only.

In reporting on cigarette use, we shall employ three perspectives (see Table 5–4). First, we examine the total population over the entire study period, reviewing the full cohort of surviving participants at each stage. Second, we report on a "core group" of patients, those who were interviewed at all four stages ($N = 205$). Finally, we review data from a panel analysis of patients, comparing responses of the individual patients at different points in time ($N = 205$).

Cigarette Smoking in Longitudinal Perspective

As Table 5–4 shows, the patients were apparently rather heavy smokers before their first heart attacks. As many as 42% smoked two packs of cigarettes or more per day, according to their own reports. Only 19% were nonsmokers. A national study in the early 1960s (Hammond & Garfinkel, 1961, 1963) reported that only 6.5% of men in the 50 to 60 year age group smoked two packs or more per day, and fully half either did not smoke at all or did so only occasionally.

With this background, the long-term performance of the study population is impressive in regard to changes in smoking behavior. At Week 7, 70% were nonsmokers, and only 4% smoked two packs or more per day. At Year 1 this sharp drop was largely being maintained; 58% reported they were nonsmokers. And at Year 8 the pattern of Year 1 persisted; 62% of survivors reported they were nonsmokers. The percentage distributions in

Table 5-4. Cigarette Smoking Level at Four Stages:
Prior to First Heart Attack and at
Week 7, Year 1, and Year 8. By Percent
of Total Population and Core Population.

Number of Cigarettes Per Day	Total Population at Each Stage			
	Prior to First Heart Attack (N = 345)	Week 7 (N = 345)	Year 1 (N = 293)	Year 8 (N = 205)
0	19.4	69.8	58.4	61.9
1-9	2.6	8.3	7.1	7.3
10	1.4	5.0	6.9	2.9
11-19	2.7	2.9	4.4	2.0
20	19.1	7.6	11.3	8.8
21-39	13.1	2.6	5.8	11.2
40-59	31.0	3.5	5.7	5.4
60 or more	10.7	.3	.4	.5
Total Percent	100.0	100.0	100.0	100.0

Number of Cigarettes Per Day	Core Population at Each Stage (N = 205)			
	Prior to First Heart Attack	Week 7	Year 1	Year 8
0	22.0	71.2	59.0	61.9
1-9	2.9	9.3	4.9	7.3
10	1.5	3.9	8.8	2.9
11-19	3.4	2.4	5.8	2.0
20	15.1	8.3	10.2	8.8
21-39	13.7	2.9	4.9	11.2
40-59	31.2	2.0	6.4	5.4
60 or more	10.2	0	0	.5
Total Percent	100.0	100.0	100.0	100.0

Source: Croog and Richards, 1977.

144

Table 5–4 are essentially the same for both the total population and for the core group.

Much current interest in the scientific and popular literature centers on the relation between smoking and mortality (Rogot, 1974; USDHEW, 1971). Although our data are not suited to the formal epidemiological analysis this issue requires, the question of smoking and subsequent death is relevant in regard to the effect of case attrition upon our findings. Thus, we may ask at Year 8 whether the reduction in smoking in our data is attributable to a higher death rate among men who were pre-illness heavy smokers.

During the full period of the study to Year 8, 79 deaths from heart disease occurred among men for whom we have smoking data. Comparing those who died with those who survived to Year 8, we examined pre-illness smoking pattern. No statistically significant differences were found.

Over the long term, the massive reduction in smoking level is apparent in all categories of smokers. This may be seen in Table 5–5 where we compare the pre-illness reports of the individual patients with their own current smoking level at Year 8.

As might be expected, the highest proportions of nonsmokers at Year 8 appear among those men who had been the lightest smokers before their first hospitalization for heart disease. But even among those men who had smoked two or more packs a day before the first infarction, considerable proportions were either nonsmokers or light smokers at Year 8. In fact, half the former "three-pack-a-day" men were now nonsmokers or smoked less than half a pack. Nearly 60% of those with a "two-pack-a-day" record were now nonsmokers or used half a pack or less at Year 8.

Thus, a fundamental and persistent change appears to have taken place in an important area of health-related behavior. Given the mixed success of smoking reduction programs for large populations, what can account for these results? One way to approach this question is to examine factors associated with patterns of smoking at selected points in time. Another is through direct examination of factors which may be associated with change and stability in level of smoking.

In an effort to develop insights on this important question, we carried out exploratory analyses using both methods. The

Table 5-5. Year 8 Smoking Level by Pre-Illness Smoking Level

Patients Smoking Given Number of Cigarettes at Year 8: by Number Smoked Prior to First Heart Attack

Number of Cigarettes Smoked Per Day Prior to First Heart Attack	Number of Cigarettes Smoked Per Day at Year 8								Total N	Percent
	None	1-9	10	11-19	20	21-39	40-59	60 or more		
None	97.8 (44)	–	–	–	2.2 (1)	–	–	–	45	100.0
1-19	68.7 (11)	6.3 (1)	12.5 (2)	–	12.5 (2)	–	–	–	16	100.0
20	61.3 (19)	9.7 (3)	3.2 (1)	6.5 (2)	9.7 (3)	6.5 (2)	3.2 (1)	–	31	100.0
21-39	50.0 (14)	10.7 (3)	7.1 (2)	–	17.9 (5)	14.3 (4)	–	–	28	100.0
40-59	48.4 (31)	9.4 (6)	1.6 (1)	1.6 (1)	7.8 (5)	21.8 (14)	9.4 (6)	–	64	100.0
60 or more	38.1 (8)	9.5 (2)	–	4.8 (1)	9.5 (2)	14.2 (3)	19.1 (4)	4.8 (1)	21	100.0
Total N	127	15	6	4	18	23	11	1	205	

principal variables examined in relation to smoking level and change were those we have already noted, including age, occupational level, educational level, and psychological self-ratings. We also considered the effects of past and present health status, based on several measures of morbidity. Finally, we included variables suggested by the Health Belief Model, such as perception of smoking as having a role in the etiology of the heart attack, perception of susceptibility and threat, belief in the efficacy of preventive action, and related items (Hochbaum, 1958; Kegeles, 1963; Rosenstock, 1974). (See Note 6 for detailed information on questions and coding.)

First, our analysis of possible correlates of smoking pattern was carried out for the data reported as of four stages: the pre-illness period and for Week 7, Year 1, and Year 8. At each stage, smoking level was not found to be significantly associated with demographic, social and psychological variables examined (Croog & Richards, 1977).

Although educational level has been linked to amount of cigarette smoking by a number of investigators (Jenkins, Zyzanski, & Rosenman, 1973; USDHEW, 1970), our data did not support such findings. However, some differences in socioeconomic level were found when we only differentiated between smokers and nonsmokers. The data indicate a negative relationship between pre-illness smoking, and both educational level and occupational level. For example, 70% of patients with some college smoked prior to their illness, while the comparable figure was 90.5% for the lowest educational group, those with 9 years of schooling or less. When occupational groups were compared in regard to smoking versus nonsmoking, the finding was similar.[8]

When we examined change and stability in smoking patterns of individuals in relation to the series of demographic, social, and psychological variables, no consistent significant relationships were found. Comparisons were made between pre-illness smoking patterns, and those at Year 1 and Year 8. These procedures were carried out primarily to fulfill the logic of the analysis, and they proved to be an exercise with predictable results. Reduction in smoking was so marked in the study population that there remained relatively few individuals who smoked at the same level or had increased their smoking. Hence, given the limited numbers of the stable smokers and "increasers," the opportunity for finding factors associated with variation or stability in pattern with this population was minimal.

It is possible, of course, that demographic, social, and psychological variables might indeed be associated with degree of change in smoking habits, particularly in the more subtle gradations over time. Limited numbers, however, precluded systematic analysis in this direction.

Smoking and the Condition of "No Further Negotiation with Fate"

Thus, we are unable to account for the marked reduction in smoking by the heart patients in terms of the demographic, social, and psychological variables we have examined. These findings of minimal correlates are consistent with the large body of data on compliance behavior which points up the still fluid state of knowledge concerning factors which predict behavior.

Nevertheless, it is easy enough to conjecture on the matter, and to offer alternative hypotheses as explanations. We might conjecture, for example, that the perceived severity of the illness over time or its degree of "threat" led to reduction in smoking. We could then anticipate finding that men with multiple heart attacks or with the most severe symptoms or impairment would later be the ones most likely to change. But this assumption was not borne out. Or, one might hypothesize that those currently with *fewest* symptoms and lowest illness level were the ones who had changed most, assuming that their minimal illness is a function of past smoking reduction. But this line of reasoning also was not supported by the data.

After Week 7, the best predictor of smoking behavior was previous smoking behavior. At Year 1 smoking level was related significantly to smoking level at Week 7. Similarly, Year 1 smoking level serves in a sense as a predictor of smoking level at Year 8. In this limited context, therefore, past smoking pattern can be interpreted as a "predictor" of future behavior. This conclusion does not hold, however, in the case of pre-illness smoking behavior. This was not related to the Week 7 posthospitalization smoking pattern.

Of all the possible influences we have reviewed, therefore, the stongest may be the fact of the illness itself. These men, previously well and living their usual lives, were afflicted with a first myocardial infarction. With this event they were transformed into persons who necessarily were aware of their continuing vulnerability, their chronic disease status, and the potentially debilitating and possibly instantly lethal nature of the disease.

It was in this context that they were advised by their physicians to give up or reduce smoking. The advice was reinforced in many ways by information in the media, antismoking programs, and folklore. The patients were thus aware that as far as smoking was concerned, there was limited further opportunity to "negotiate with fate." The choice was to reduce or give up smoking—or to experience an unpleasant alternative. Though reducing smoking might not prevent subsequent heart attacks, the risks associated with smoking perhaps appeared more clear-cut to these patients with a potentially lethal illness than they would to other persons.

Some further clues to the role of perceived immediate vulnerability in smoking reduction can be seen in the record of smoking by the patients' wives (Croog & Richards, 1977). Wives were interviewed at Week 7 and Year 1, and data were collected in regard to their smoking behavior as well as their beliefs and attitudes regarding etiology, prevention, and control of heart disease.

The data show that the wives did not differ from their husbands in regard to beliefs about the role of smoking in the etiology of heart disease, or the preventive effects of smoking reduction. But even while their husbands reduced or gave up smoking during Year 1, the wives continued to smoke, showing no change from their pattern before the husband's illness.

A main difference, we suggest, is that the threat of death and disability from heart disease was less immediate for the wives than for the husbands. Though such events might be in prospect, they were far off in the future, and possibly they might never happen at all. In other words, the wives perceived they still had the possibility for "negotiation with fate," for taking a chance on smoking, and for avoiding the distant illness.

Summary

Covering a period of 8 years, this chapter has centered on two aspects of patient compliance with the medical regimen: compliance orientation and reported compliance behavior.

Of patients who reported receiving physician advice in any of 10 principal areas at Year 8, a majority reported positive compliance orientation on six: medications, work, rest, exercise, alcohol consumption, and sexual activity. Positive compliance orientation was strongest with regard to medications.

Among those patients who reported receiving physician advice, the proportion with positive compliance orientation declined over time from Week 7 to Year 8. Use of medications was the only exception to this trend. It was suggested that the decreased positive compliance orientation over the 8 years might reflect a lessening in feelings of urgency about the illness and/or gradual adoption of a more flexible attitude toward medical advice.

Few consistent patterns of statistical association emerged at Year 8 between compliance orientation toward individual items of physician advice and selected socioeconomic variables, psychological self-rating traits, conceptions of the etiology of the disease, or measures of health status. However, age of patients was positively related to compliance with physician advice on alcohol consumption, weight control, dietary practices, and use of medications. With regard to advice on smoking, exercise, weight control, diet, and use of medications, positive compliance orientation at Week 7 and/or Year 1 was subsequently associated with positive orientation at Year 8.

Cigarette smoking by the patients was examined as an example of reported compliance behavior over time. In comparison with the pre-illness period, cigarette use declined sharply by Week 7. This reduction appears evident also at the end of the 8-year period. It constitutes one relatively unusual example of long-term change in smoking behavior within a sizeable study population. As possible correlates of change in smoking level, we examined demographic, social, and psychological variables, as well as severity of illness and health beliefs. No significant associations emerged.

A possible factor underlying change in patient smoking behavior may have been recognition of the impending and unpredictable threat of subsequent heart attacks and death. There thus was little further possibility for rationalizing smoking or for "negotiating with fate."

NOTES

1.   As the literature in this area points out, there are a number of variables which might bear on the problem:

   a.   characteristics of the advice—specificity, difficulty, deprivation involved, costs, time investment required, and the like.
   b.   characteristics of the physician—professional background, training, social characteristics, psychological traits, position in status systems (the medical profession, hospital, community social structure) and the like.
   c.   characteristics of the patient—social characteristics, psychological traits, position in status systems, nature of illness, view of illness, experience in medical sphere (preprogramming), attitudes (view of authority, importance attributed to health), and the like.
   d.   characteristics of communication and communication process— mode of delivery, timing, emotional tone, structure, and content of interaction system between doctor and patient.
   e.   social structural elements and content of social setting—factors in environment affecting compliance, such as group norms, family norms, work situation, and the like.

2.   With regard to the relationship between favorable orientation toward compliance and actual performance, Kegeles reports on a study of motivation to be examined for cervical cancer. Although not a perfect predictor, the best indicator of subsequent follow-through in obtaining a cytological examination was stated intention to do so. Those who stated negative or ambivalent intentions usually did not have the examination. See Kegeles, 1967.

3.   Twenty men who reported receiving no physician advice on any of the selected items were excluded from crosstabulations using the C-O Index.

4.   Selected independent variables used in the analysis of correlates of compliance orientation were coded as follows:

  a. Age at Week 7: (1) 30 to 34; (2) 35 to 39; (3) 40 to 44; (4) 45 to 49; (5) 50 to 54; and (6) 55 to 60.
  b. Educational level: (1) 1 year of college or more; (2) high school diploma; and (3) less than high school diploma.
  c. Pre-illness occupational level: (1) executive and professional; (2) upper white-collar; (3) lower white-collar; (4) skilled blue-collar; and (5) semiskilled and unskilled blue-collar.
  d. Self-rated psychological characteristics "feelings easily hurt," "bossy," "easily depressed," "in a hurry," "ambitious," "eats rapidly,": (1) not at all; (2) a little or somewhat; and (3) considerably or very much.
  e. Total number of symptoms experienced at Year 8: (1) none; (2) 1 to 4; (3) 5 to 6; (4) 7 to 8; (5) 9 or more.
  f. Selected symptoms, including "breathlessness," "heart skipping beat," and "sleeplessness" reported in the month prior to the Year 8 interview: (1) not at all; (2) once or twice; and (3) three times or more.
  g. Self-described health at Year 8: (1) excellent; (2) very good; (3) good; and (4) fair to poor.
  h. Number of days spent in bed in the year prior to the Year 8 interview: (1) none; (2) 5 or fewer; and (3) 6 to 26.
  i. Number of consultations of a doctor in the year prior to the Year 8 interview: (1) none; (2) 1; (3) 2 to 5; (4) 6 to 10; and (5) 11 or more.
  j. Physician rating at Year 8 of patient's cardiac status coded as (1) uncompromised; (2) slightly compromised; and (3) moderately to severely compromised.
  k. Physician's assessment of patient's cardiac prognosis at Year 8: (1) good; (2) good with therapy; (3) fair with therapy; and (4) guarded.
  l. Physician's rating of patient's functional health status at Year 8: (1) no significant impairment; (2) moderate impairment; and (3) severe impairment.
  m. Number of heart-related hospitalizations since Year 1: (1) rehospitalized for heart; (2) rehospitalized for other reasons; and (3) not rehospitalized.

  n. Compliance orientation on individual items (work, rest, exercise, smoking, drinking, weight, diet, medications, avoiding quarrels) at Week 7 and Year 1: (1) complete compliance; (2) other.

  o. Patient's perceptions of importance of such factors as smoking, drinking, overweight, and work tension in the etiology of his illness: (1) important; (2) not important.

  p. Previous score on the C-O Index at Week 7 and Year 1: (1) high; (2) medium; and (3) low.

5. Some materials for this section have also been reported in Croog and Richards, 1977.

6. Variables which assessed the health beliefs of the patients in relation to smoking behavior were as follows:

  a. Belief in the power of the individual: activity versus passivity. Patients were asked at Week 7, "Thinking back to the days before you became sick, are there some specific things you did which might have brought on the attack? Possible responses were "yes," "no," and "don't know."

  b. Belief in the power of the individual: possibility of preventive action. Patients were asked at Week 7, "Before you became sick, what things do you think you could have done to help avoid having the attack?" The possible responses were "nothing," "something," and "don't know." To assess patients' perceptions of personal control over future events, they were asked at Year 1, "Do you feel there is anything you can do to prevent getting sick again?"

  c. Perceptions of susceptibility: symptoms and rehospitalization. Patients were asked at Week 7, Year 1, and Year 8, "During the past month, how often have you had pain or discomfort such as the following?" Symptoms included chest pain, breathlessness, heart pounding, getting tired easily, and other symptoms commonly associated with heart disease. The possible responses were "none," and "only occasionally," fairly often," "very often," and "don't know." Data on number of rehospitalizations and reasons for admission were obtained from the patients at Year 1 and Year 8 and from their physicians at Year 1.

7. Chi-square = 11.50, d.f. = 3, $p < .01$, gamma = .31.

8. Chi-square = 13.74, d.f. = 3, $p < .01$, gamma = .38.

Chapter 6

PATIENTS AND THEIR FAMILIES

Life with Illness

INTRODUCTION

Among the central elements in the "armory of resources" are the social supports provided to a patient by his family and kin network. A constructive and supportive response to the illness by family members, the emotional quality of relationships with wives and children, and the types of services and aid provided by family and quasi-kin may play a significant part in how the patient handles his illness.

It is widely recognized that the presence of serious, chronic illness in a family member can have pervasive effects on relationships within the family. As Litman (1974) points out, "Apparently, in the face of such strain, familial cohesion is subject to the severest test, with the outcome left very much in doubt." However, systematic documentation of these effects of chronic illness on the family is relatively rare.

In this chapter we examine several aspects of family life in the context of illness. In doing so, we report on patients' perceptions of the effects of their illness on other family members, the influence of the illness on the employment of wives, and some elements of the relationship between husband and wife. We also examine patients' perceptions of involvement of family members in the etiology of their illness, and the roles of kin and quasi-kin groups as sources of social support.

In considering illness and family life, a salient feature of the health history of the study population should be noted once again. As we reported in Chapter 2, there was considerable variation in the amount of illness which the men experienced over the 8 years. Some patients, indeed, had no recurrence of acute illness after their first heart attack, and they lived relatively uneventful lives, as far as their health was concerned. Others, as we have seen, were more severely affected. As a group, however, the men in the study population shared a common characteristic: all were afflicted by a progressive and chronic disease. Thus, in one way or another, patients had to confront the daily reality of being persons with heart disease, and in one way or another, their families had to cope with this fact as well.

FAMILY STRUCTURE AND COMPOSITION OF THE HOME

As background to our report, let us briefly review some principal features of the patients' marriages and family arrangements. In the period from Year 1 to Year 8, the marital situations of the patients remained relatively stable. A high proportion of the men (88%) were married at the time of Year 8, nearly all (95%) to the same women who were their wives at Year 1. Eighty-two percent of the total group were living with their wives, and about half of these also had children in their homes. A small number—6%—were living alone. The remainder of the population lived in various combinations of household arrangements with wives, children, and other relatives. Thus, the population as a whole is charactarized by high stability in marriage and types of living arrangements common to the American scene.

LIVING WITH ILLNESS: PERCEIVED EFFECTS ON FAMILY MEMBERS

In chronic, life-threatening illness, the burdens and stresses associated with the disease often fall not only on the patient but on other members of the household as well. After a period of approximately 8 years following the first heart attack, how does the patient perceive the impact of his illness on other family members?

This question is an exceedingly difficult one to explore, for it deals with complex and often subtle interpersonal phenomena, the perception of these phenomena, and the ways in which a patient is able or willing to conceptualize and report them in a survey-research-type interview. Further, the unconscious mechanism of denial may operate, serving as a means of coping with the illness and with associated stress and suffering among other family members. Hence, although there may be considerable stresses within the family, the patient may report they are not present.

Our examination of the patient-reported impact of the illness on other family members centers primarily on responses to two related questions, "In what main ways do you think your illness has affected your wife?" and "In what main ways do you think your illness has affected your children living at home?"

Responses to these questions were examined in relation to measures of health status of the patients at Year 8. These include assessments by their physicians in terms of several perspectives: (1) current cardiac status, (2) cardiac prognosis, (3) functional health status, and (4) major medical and surgical problems which significantly handicap the patient in his health and functioning. Another measure of relative morbidity is the history of one or more rehospitalizations during the period since Year 1. (For further discussion, see Chapters 2 and 8 and Appendix C.)

Perceived Effects on Wives and Children

How did the patients view the impact of their illness on their families? Were their perceptions related to their health status? Among married patients responding (N = 180), 63% cited some effects of the illness on their wives. Among patients with children living at home (N = 95), 33% cited effects on their children.

Data concerning patients' perceptions of the effects of their illness (cardiac or other) on their wives and children can be seen in Table 6–1. As we would expect, the most severely ill men reported in highest proportions concerning the effects of illness on spouses and children. However, of perhaps equal interest is the proportion of patients with the most favorable health ratings

Table 6-1. Reported Perception by Patient That His Illness Had Effects
on His Wife and Children. By Health Status at Year 8[*]

Measure of Health Status	Illness Had Effects on Wife		Illness Had Effects on Children	
	Number of Patients	Percent	Number of Patients	Percent
Cardiac Status				
Uncompromised	38/58	65.5	6/28	21.4
Slightly compromised	24/39	61.5	5/16	31.3
Moderately or severely compromised	22/26	84.6	9/11	81.8
Cardiac Prognosis				
Good	39/58	67.2	6/23	26.1
Good with therapy	17/33	51.5	6/17	35.3
Fair or guarded despite therapy	28/34	82.4	8/16	50.0
Functional Health Status				
No significant impairment	51/79	64.6	10/37	27.0
Moderate or severe impairment	30/40	75.0	9/17	53.0
Major Illness or Condition Impairing Health and Functioning				
Absent	21/36	58.3	4/17	23.5
Present	63/90	70.0	17/40	42.5
Rehospitalization Year 1 – Year 8				
Not rehospitalized since Year 1	42/68	61.8	12/38	31.6
Hospitalized in other than previous 2 years	31/49	63.3	7/26	26.9
Hospitalized in previous 2 years	37/54	68.5	11/23	47.8

[*]The first four measures of health status are derived from physicians' ratings, unavailable for some patients for varying reasons (See Note 2, Chapter 2). Physician ratings were reported for 72% of married patients and 66% of patients with at-home children at Year 8.

who also report negative effects. They include, for example, about two-thirds of the men with uncompromised cardiac status and good cardiac prognosis. Given our recognition of the operation of the denial mechanism, we can assume that the reported perceptions in the table provide only a minimal estimate.

A perhaps more interesting feature of the table involves

perceived effects of the illness on wives as compared with children. In general, the most severely ill patients reported their wives as somewhat more affected than their children. However, the differences are most marked in the case of the *least* ill. These men perceived the impact of their illness on their wives as markedly greater than on their children. These data may indicate that the patients see their wives as concerned even though they appear to be relatively well, but see their children as concerned only if they are moderately or severely compromised.

Some indications of the nature of perceived impact of the illness upon wives and children are provided by patient descriptions. Patients who reported effects were asked to specify them. The relative ranking of their responses is shown in Table 6-2.

Increased anxiety and concern was the primary reported effect on patients' wives. Next most common was increased protectiveness and care of the patient. As examples, patients de-

Table 6-2. Reported Effects of Patients' Illness on Wives: Patients' Perceptions

Reported Effect	Number of Patients (Base N = 175*)	Percent
Increase in Wife's Anxiety, Worry, and Insecurity	66	37.7
Increased in Wife's Protectiveness and Care of Patient	36	20.6
Changes in Diet, Menu, or Cooking Patterns	17	9.7
Increase in Wife's Responsibility for Household and Family Maintenance	14	8.0
Increase or Reduction in Wife's Paid Employment	14	8.0
Changes in Style of Life or Spending Patterns	5	2.9
Reduction in Wife's Social and Recreational Activities	3	1.7
Other	14	8.0

*Married patients only. Percentages are not cumulative as some patients gave multiple responses.

scribed their wives as seeing to it that they followed the physician's regimen, and helping them to avoid conflict in the home, such as confrontations with the children. Relatively few reported changes in roles or responsibilities in the home which they ascribed to the illness. Least often noted were changes in the wife's social activities. Judging by this series of rankings, the primary perceived impact on the wives appears to be emotional, while effects on life style and social participation were minimal.

As noted earlier, only a third of the patients with children at home perceived them as having been affected by the illness. Although the numbers are small, the data suggest several themes. As in the case of the wives, the perceived effects on children were primarily emotional. There were few indications of perceived effects on education, social activities, life plans, or other matters.

In considering the long-term influence of the illness on family life, we can look back at earlier reports by the patients concerning their wives and children. At Year 1, for example, 73% of married patients cited effects of the illness on their wives, compared to 63% in the cohort at Year 8. The specific effects reported at Year 1 ranked substantially the same as at Year 8. At Year 1, furthermore, 55% of patients with children at home noted effects, as compared to 33% at Year 8. Again, the general pattern of ranking of effects was similar to that at Year 8.

Within some families it is evident that similar basic concerns were present at both Year 1 and at Year 8. Among those men who noted increased anxiety among their wives at Year 8 in association with the illness, 56% had made similar observations at Year 1. Similarly, among those who reported an increase in protectiveness in their wives at Year 8, 36% reported it 7 years earlier.

Our assessment of these data must be tempered with qualifications, of course. For example, the health status of the men at Year 8 was distinctive in many ways from that at Year 1, and the causes for concern were thus different. However, the data imply a continuity of problems in some families, pinpointing a subgroup in this patient population which was especially burdened by problems of anxiety and insecurity in the wives over the years. Such men and their families might thus constitute a special target population which might benefit from supportive services and counsel.

IMPACT OF THE ILLNESS ON THE HOME: THE EMPLOYMENT OF WIVES

Among the changes which sometimes occur as a result of illness are changes in the employment status of spouses. Long-term, chronic illness sometimes makes it necessary to enlist another source of support for the home, especially if the patient is principal or sole "breadwinner." In Chapter 3, we reported briefly on patients' wives in the work force. Here we shall consider effects of their employment on relationships within the family.

As we noted earlier, among the married couples at Year 8, 54% of the wives were employed. In our study population, heart disease in the husband was not generally affecting marriages by causing wives to go to work or to remain employed. In fact, illness of the husband influenced the current employment of wives in only about 14% of all couples.

On the whole, at Year 8 the benefits of employment of the wives far outweighed the possible disadvantages. As many as 88% of the men with working wives reported no problems at all associated with their spouses' employment. The rest primarily reported negative effects upon the marital relationship. However, perceptions of the wife's employment as a source of marital problems were not particularly greater in those families where her working was motivated by the husband's illness. These findings were similar to those we reported in our earlier study concerning Year 1.

ILLNESS IN OTHER FAMILY MEMBERS: THE STRESSOR TRIGGER HYPOTHESIS AT YEAR 8

As we saw in Chapter 2, the burdens of illness had become familiar to many patients by Year 8. Two-thirds had been rehospitalized over the years, and many were now described by their physicians as having medical problems which might significantly handicap their adjustment or functioning. For a number of these patients, however, the problems of their own illness were also exacerbated by serious illness in other members of the household. This situation helped complicate the patients' ability to cope by adding emotional strain and, in some cases, financial stress.

In 31% of the homes, at least one person other than the patient was reported as having an illness and/or continuing chronic health condition during the previous year.[1] In two-thirds of these cases, the illnesses were "major," i.e., life threatening and/or seriously disabling. The remainder were minor illnesses. Very minor ailments such as the common cold, upset stomach, and simple abrasions or cuts and the like are excluded from this analysis. In most of these households (70%), at least one of the ill persons was the wife. Next in rank were homes in which a child was ill, followed by a small percentage of households with a sick parent or other relative.

The number of patients who reported heart disease in other family members was relatively small. Seven percent of the wives ($N = 14$) were described as having some type of heart disease or circulatory disorder, and only four patients were living with a parent, child, or other family member with heart disease.[2]

It has sometimes been suggested that illness of one family member may serve as a stressor trigger leading to illness in other family members. In our study, however, no association was found between level of illness of the patients and the total burden of illness in the home. We pursued the issue in various ways. A series of crosstabulations was made, examining differing measures of morbidity in patients in relation to total burden of illness in the home, and in relation to presence or absence of serious illness in the wife during the previous year. No significant statistical relationships appeared. For example, when we look at total illness burden in the home, the households of men who were most severely impaired by heart disease did not differ from those of moderately impaired or unimpaired men. A similar finding had emerged at Year 1, as reported in our earlier work.

ILLNESS AND THE MARITAL RELATIONSHIP: HAPPINESS AND DISAGREEMENT

There is considerable speculation and much conflicting evidence about the effects of illness and its accompanying stresses upon the quality of the marriage relationship (Aguilera & Messick, 1974; Litman, 1974). It has been suggested, for example,

that severe, life-threatening illness serves to draw marital partners closer together. Some have postulated that the stresses of
illness are essentially disruptive and tend to damage the marital
relationship. Still another view is that illness makes little difference in the basic dynamics of the relationship and that more
deeply rooted factors are important. Patients' responses concerning marital happiness and marital disagreement may offer some
insights into this complex issue in our study population.

In the Year 8 interview, married men were asked to rate their
own marital happiness and that of their wives. Half considered
themselves to be "very happily married" (49.5%). A third of the
men described their marriages as "happy" but chose not to characterize themselves as "very happily" married. Fifteen percent
called their marriages "average," and 2% termed them "unhappy" or "very unhappy." Their reports on how they perceived the
marital happiness of their wives were similar: 46% "very happy,"
35% "happy," 16% "average," and 3% "unhappy" or "very unhappy."

Although these data can be examined in many ways, the
relevant issue here is the relationship of marital happiness to
illness level. Crosstabulations show that the reported degree of
marital happiness at Year 8 was not related to the patient's health
status, as assessed by the various indices of morbidity.

The interview at Year 8 also included a series of 12 questions
probing major areas of disagreement between the patient and his
wife. The items were based in part on the Burgess and Wallin
measures of marital disagreement (1953).[3] The total number of
items reported by the husband served as his score on an index
ranging from 0 to 7 or more. As in the case of the marital
happiness items, the marital disagreement score was examined in
relation to measures of morbidity. We found that the level of
reported marital disagreement did not differ significantly by the
level of severity of the patient's illness, as measured by the health
status indices described earlier.

Patients' rankings of areas of disagreement at Year 8 were
similar to rankings at Year 1. As at Year 1, the items most frequently cited as points of disagreement at Year 8 were "handling
family finances" (34%), "how to spend leisure time" (34%), and
"bringing up children" (31%).

The only individual area of disagreement related to severity of illness in the husband at Year 8 was "handling family finances." The men categorized as most impaired by the five measures of severity listed in Table 6-1 appeared *least* likely to disagaree with their wives on finances. For example, 11% of those patients whose physician-rated cardiac status was moderately or severely compromised cited finances as an area of disagreement, while 40% of those with "uncompromised" cardiac status did so (chi square = 7.21, d.f. = 2, $p < .05$). The reasons for this pattern are not clear, and the results may be only a product of statistical random variation. However, the data may also reflect changes in role relations in the home and perhaps a tendency for the most ill men to accept their wives' management of finances.

The most useful predictor of a couple's total pattern of reported marital happiness and marital disagreement at Year 8 was their happiness and disagreement at Year 1. Responses of each patient at Year 1 were crosstabulated with his responses at Year 8, provided he was still married to the same woman. The gamma correlation between measures of marital happiness was .50. For reported marital disagreement, the mean gamma score for all 12 items was .66.

PROTECTIVE RESTRICTIONS BY PATIENTS' WIVES

Another potential influence of illness upon the home is that it may alter mutual nurturing or protective responses of marital partners. In the case of heart disease in males, such changes may take the form of efforts by patients' wives to restrict their activities and to limit the stresses upon them. Patients were asked at Year 8, "Has your wife made attempts to keep you from doing more than you should?" Four-fifths (81%) of the married men responded in the affirmative.

One of the interesting aspects of this response involves the question of its relationship to the patients' level of illness. When we examined wives' reported protective response in relation to our measures of severity of illness in the patient at Year 8, we found no statistically significant relationships. Indeed, men who were least ill reported in the same proportions as did others that their wives acted protectively.

There were significant associations between patients' earlier reports of their wives' protectiveness at Week 7 and Year 1 and responses at Year 8. Of those men with the same wives who responded positively at Year 8, 85% had also reported affirmatively at Week 7 and at Year 1 with regard to their wives' efforts to restrict them. The gamma correlations between responses at Year 1 and Year 8 and between Week 7 and Year 8 were .57 and .81, respectively. It seems, then, that the character of the long-term marital relationship rather than the immediate severity of illness may better explain the wife's efforts to protect or restrict her husband.

Those men who were the most severely ill responded in somewhat higher proportions that one way in which their wives protected or restricted them was by assuming some of their former duties in the household. For example, 32.4% of those rated as impaired, compared with 21% of the unimpaired, reported that their wives had taken over some of their duties. However, these differences are not statistically significant. In this case, level of illness does not appear to be the crucial variable in determining the "adoption" of the husband's duties by the wife.

Approximately half the married men (55%) indicated that their wives believed that they were not sufficiently careful in regard to their health. Of this group, 17% also stated that their wives had taken over some of their former duties. However, among those who responded that their wives perceived them as "about right" in the way they took care of their health, 19% also reported the assumption of their duties by their wives.

Considering the issue of change in role relationships, two principal points may be noted here. First, a majority of the men, even including the most impaired, still perceived themselves as maintaining the roles they had performed before the onset of their illness. Second, although they were in reasonably good health, about one-fifth of the "unimpaired" husbands nevertheless perceived their wives as taking over their duties. Of course, we are reporting here solely on perceptions by one marital partner, and denial and other emotional factors may affect such perceptions. However, these data imply that even in many cases of relatively well men, the illness may provide a trigger and justification for a shift in power relations between husband and wife.

In sum, these materials on the influence of illness upon family life appear to reflect complex processes in other spheres of relationships as well. Level of marital happiness, marital disagreement, and perceived degree of protective restrictions by wives are not related in a simplistic way to severity of the husbands' illness, but rather they appear to be more strongly influenced by deeper, long-term processes. The data perhaps reaffirm that how husband and wife have related to each other over the course of years may be more of an influence upon their current lives than the illness itself. Indeed, in some cases, assumption of the husband's duties by the wife appears to illustrate that the illness may only provide a context for working out of continuing strains for power, authority, and dominance.

ASCRIBING BLAME TO WIFE AND CHILDREN: AN HISTORICAL VIEW OF PERCEPTION OF ETIOLOGY

Indications of the emotional meaning of the illness in the home can sometimes be gained by probing patients' beliefs concerning etiology. As we have noted earlier, patients were asked in the Year 8 interview to rate in importance a series of 17 possible etiological factors which might have caused their heart attacks. The items included various physical, social, psychological, and interpersonal factors (Koslowsky, Croog, & La Voie, 1978). Two are relevant here: "upsetting problems with children" and "problems with wife."

Nearly one out of five married men at Year 8 (18.8%) reported that problems with their wives were either somewhat or very important in the etiology of the heart attack. No differences were found between the perceptions of men who had been most recently hospitalized for heart disease, and those who remained "well" for the entire period since Year 8. There were no statistically significant differences in perceptions between men of differing social status levels, educational backgrounds, or occupational groups.

In the case of men who had children, the situation was analogous in many respects. Here, 16% at Year 8 stated that upsetting problems with their children had contributed to the etiology of the heart attack. There was a major difference from the data concerning wives, however; patients varied in response by health level. Among those men who had been rehospitalized for heart disease since Year 1, 30% cited problems with their children as causes. Among those men who had not been rehospitalized for cardiac reasons, only 11% cited their children. The findings were similar for other measures of morbidity since Year 1. For example, those men rated as impaired by their physicians reported in significantly higher proportions that their children had helped cause the heart attack.

Patients' perceptions at Year 8 of the role of family members in causing their heart attacks are consistent with those reported during the first year. At Week 7, 18% of the married men cited problems with their wives, and 25% of those with children cited problems with their children as important in the etiology of their illness. At Year 1, the proportions were similar to those at Week 7. In sum, the perceptions as reported by the cohort at each interview stage remained relatively static over time.

Perhaps of more consequence to our consideration of the impact of the illness on the family is the persistence of these beliefs among the same respondents. Indeed, when we compare the responses of the men at Year 8 with their own reports at Week 7, it appears that nearly half of those who cited their wives at Week 7 continued to do so at Year 8. Similarly, of those who cited problems with their children as important at Week 7, one-third continued to do so at Year 8.

Moreover, earlier data suggest that the husbands were not alone in such views. At Year 1, for example, 22% of wives ($N = 226$) mentioned "problems with wife," and 26% ($N = 216$) of those wives with children mentioned "problems with children" as important etiological factors. Not all the husbands and wives who cited these factors were married to each other. In 37% of the marriages at Year 1, the husband, the wife, or both mentioned the wife's role in etiology. Thus, in over one-third of marriages at that time, one or both spouses indicated a belief that the wife had some part in causing the heart attack. A similar point can be made about the number of families in which either one or both parents expressed beliefs about the etiological effect of conflict involving their children.

Since some respondents may have been reluctant to answer

affirmatively on these sensitive questions, it is likely that an even greater proportion felt that problems with the wives and children contributed to the illness. The cardiovascular system is highly sensitive to changes in emotional state, but we can only conjecture about the effects of recrimination, accusation, guilt, and silent aggression implied by the expressed beliefs. Whether or not such perceptions ascribing "blame" have a real impact on the long-term physical course of the disease, they unquestionably color relationships within the home and affect how the patient and family deal with the illness.

SOURCES OF SUPPORT AND AID: LONG-TERM PERSPECTIVES

Two important elements in the repertoire of support systems of the heart patients were: (1) the extended kin group, and (2) non-family members such as friends and neighbors functioning in a "quasi-kin" role (Croog, Lipson, & Levine, 1972).[4] In order that we might explore the contributions made by both types of resources, we asked patients at Year 8 to rate the degree of help they received from various categories of both kin and non-kin during the previous year.[5]

Perceived Helpfulness

When we examined the total population without regard to illness status at Year 8, some interesting patterns emerged. Children were a prominent source of support: in ratings of helpfulness, high proportions of patients with children cited them as helpful in some degree. However, among other possible sources, non-kin (friends and neighbors) were nearly as important on the whole as close kin such as parents and siblings. Virtually all patients reported receiving help of some sort during the previous year. Only 3% indicated that no one from among the sources listed had helped them. (See Table 6-3).

One variable affecting use of support sources is obviously "need," and the severity of illness may be one of the salient indicators of possible need. Do the most severely ill patients differ from the "healthiest" in use of kin and non-kin resources? This

Table 6-3. Degree of Help From Kin and Non-Kin Reported at Year 8

Source of Help	Number of Patients Reporting Help*	Degree of Help					
		Very Helpful		Somewhat or Not Too Helpful		Not at All Helpful	
		N	Percent	N	Percent	N	Percent
Kin							
Parents	57	18	31.6	17	29.8	22	38.6
Children	171	91	53.2	53	31.0	27	15.8
Siblings	171	41	24.0	58	33.9	72	42.1
In-Laws	172	43	25.0	49	28.5	80	46.5
Other Relatives	144	18	12.5	43	29.9	83	57.6
Non-Kin							
Friends	197	56	28.4	72	36.6	69	35.0
Neighbors	196	42	21.4	73	37.3	81	41.3

*"Not relevant" and "don't know" responses have been omitted.

question was approached in part through use of various measures of health status (number of symptoms, rehospitalization history, number of physician visits in the preceding year, and physicians' ratings of functional health status). Our findings are presented in Table 6-4.

As Table 6-4 shows, those with the least favorable health status did not report substantially greater support than those with the most favorable record. Although there are some minor variations, the general patterning is similar on all the health status measures shown. Contrary to expectation, in some instances those with the poorest health indicators reported in lowest proportions that a source had been helpful to them.

Non-kin resources appear also as important sources of aid for all groups, matching the various kin categories in frequency of mention. Even among those who were the least ill, high proportions noted various types of non-kin sources as helpful to them in the previous year. For example, among those not rehospitalized since Year 1, 64% cited friends and 54% cited neighbors as helpful in some degree.

These data, of course, in part are a product of the cultural pattern of mutual aid and moral support shared by relatives, friends, and neighbors in American society (Sussman, 1969). Hence, it is not surprising that the relatively "well" patients refer in positive ways to their experiences with kin and non-kin over the past year. The more notable findings here, however, are centered in the data on men with some degree of symptoms and impairment. These men do not significantly differ from the most well men in their perceptions of the helpfulness of others in kin and non-kin groups.

We attempted to systematically evaluate the relationship between help sources and various characteristics of the patient, including age at Year 8, educational level, social class, and frequency of social visits. In the analysis of these data, level of helpfulness by the kin and non-kin sources was not related to either age or social status indicators. However, there was an association between patient visiting patterns and reported degree of help received. Patients with patterns of more frequent social visits were more likely to report help from both relatives and non-kin sources. These findings are, of course, consistent with

Table 6-4. Sources of Reported Help. By Patient's Health Status at Year 8

Measure of Health Status[/]	Source of Help*						
	Parents	Children	Siblings	In-Laws	Other Relatives	Friends	Neighbors
Number of Symptoms							
0-2	58.8 (17)	87.3 (55)	63.1 (46)	53.9 (52)	48.9 (45)	68.3 (60)	55.0 (60)
3-4	60.8 (23)	76.5 (51)	52.8 (53)	48.0 (52)	35.4 (48)	65.5 (58)	57.9 (57)
5-6	– (7/9)‡	84.3 (38)	62.5 (40)	63.9 (36)	50.0 (24)	68.2 (44)	75.0 (44)
7 or more	– (4/8)	92.6 (27)	53.2 (32)	50.0 (32)	37.0 (27)	54.3 (35)	45.7 (35)
Most Recent Hospitalization							
None since Year 1	62.5 (24)	90.5 (63)	64.4 (59)	51.6 (62)	43.4 (53)	63.9 (72)	54.2 (72)
Over 1 year	60.9 (23)	83.3 (72)	60.7 (79)	59.5 (74)	41.9 (62)	67.1 (85)	64.0 (86)
Within 1 year	– (3/6)	75.8 (33)	41.4 (29)	40.7 (32)	44.0 (25)	63.9 (36)	58.9 (34)
Visits to Physician in Preceding Year							
0-1	80.0 (15)	83.8 (37)	70.0 (40)	69.5 (36)	50.0 (28)	69.1 (42)	62.8 (43)
2-5	53.6 (28)	88.1 (84)	58.5 (77)	52.9 (87)	44.3 (70)	66.3 (95)	58.5 (94)
6-20	57.2 (14)	77.1 (48)	48.1 (52)	42.5 (47)	36.4 (44)	58.6 (58)	56.1 (57)
Physician's Rating of Functional Health Status							
No significant impairment	78.6 (28)	82.0 (78)	61.8 (76)	54.5 (77)	41.5 (65)	63.7 (91)	59.8 (87)
Moderate or severe impairment	– (1/9)	86.5 (37)	51.2 (43)	60.0 (40)	45.4 (33)	66.7 (45)	58.7 (46)

*Figures represent all degrees of reported helpfulness except "not at all helpful." Separate analyses of different degrees of helpfulness did not alter results obtained when all degrees were combined. Base N's are in parentheses.

[/]Other morbidity indicators examined were: major reasons for physician visit in past year, number of heart-related hospitalizations since Year 1, and physician rating of patient cardiac status. These were omitted from the table for reasons of brevity. Results were not different from those reported in the table.

‡In instances where the base N is less than 10, the percentage has not been computed. Both numerator and denominator are presented in parentheses in such cases.

170

common assumptions regarding social integration and receipt of aid—by definition, socially integrated people have relatives and associates who are linked to them and who will aid them.

Perhaps the more important aspect of the data, however, concerns the lack of use of supports by men with a low level of social participation. For example, 37% of the total group reported no visits with friends and these same men cited no friends as helpful. Similarly, 43% indicated neither visits with neighbors nor any helpful neighbors. This pattern is essentially no different for the rehospitalized than for the nonrehospitalized patients. It thus appears that nonreceipt of aid and support may be more the product of level of social integration of the individual than of need in a time of illness. These results at Year 8 are similar to those which we found in our earlier study of the year after the first heart attack (Croog, Lipson, & Levine, 1972).

Types of Help Reported from Kin and Non-Kin

How do kin and non-kin sources compare in terms of the *type* of assistance provided? We turn now to consider three principal categories of aid: moral support, services, and financial assistance. As Table 6-5 shows, the principal type of aid received from all sources was moral support. Services provided by neighbors and friends were reported by as high a proportion of men as reported services from members of the nuclear family. In fact, citation of services from non-kin, neighbors, and friends, was substantially larger than reports on services from "other relatives."

Table 6-5 also shows that the recently hospitalized, and the not recently hospitalized patients report similar patterns of types of support received. In other terms, in general, those with the poorest health histories report patterns of receipt of services similar to those of the healthier patient. The principal difference is in the category, receipt of aid from siblings. The recently hospitalized patients received almost twice as much moral support, but considerably less services and financial aid, from their brothers and sisters than the patients who were not recently hospitalized.

In sum, after 8 years, the role of family members as support

Table 6-5. Type of Help from Kin and Non-Kin Reported at Year 8. By Total Study Population, Recently Hospitalized and Not Recently Hospitalized

Source of Help	Number of Patients Reporting Help[*]	Type of Help[†]					
		Moral Support		Services		Financial Aid	
		N	Percent	N	Percent	N	Percent
Total Study Population							
Kin							
Parents	29	23	79.3	2	6.9	8	27.6
Children	126	76	60.3	88	69.8	10	7.9
Siblings	70	59	84.3	24	34.3	7	10.0
In-laws	65	49	75.4	25	38.5	9	13.9
Other Relatives	27	26	96.3	6	22.2	3	11.1
Non-Kin							
Friends	99	67	68.0	42	42.4	3	3.0
Neighbors	78	46	59.0	46	59.0	1	1.3
Hospitalized in Previous 2 Years							
Kin							
Parents	7[≠]	6	–	0	–	1	–
Children	36	17	47.2	16	44.4	3	8.3
Siblings	19	18	94.7	1	5.3	0	0.0
In-laws	23	13	56.5	8	34.8	2	8.7
Other Relatives	10	7	70.0	1	10.0	2	20.0
Non-Kin							
Friends	36	23	63.9	11	30.6	2	5.6
Neighbors	32	15	46.9	16	50.0	1	3.1

sources is clearly varied. Children rank foremost as sources of services, but moral support is particularly drawn from parents, siblings, in-laws, and other relatives. At the same time, surrogate or "quasi-family," as exemplified by friends and neighbors, are also of considerable importance. While severity of illness or "need

Table 6-5.   (Continued)

Source of Help	Number of Patients Reporting Help*	Type of Help†				Financial Aid	
		Moral Support		Services			
		N	Percent	N	Percent	N	Percent
Not Hospitalized in Previous 2 Years							
Kin							
Parents	21	13	61.9	2	9.5	6	28.6
Children	88	20	22.7	61	69.3	7	8.0
Siblings	51	25	49.0	19	37.3	7	13.7
In-laws	40	20	50.0	15	37.5	5	12.5
Other Relatives	17	12	70.6	4	23.5	1	5.9
Non-Kin							
Friends	62	31	50.0	30	48.4	1	1.6
Neighbors	46	16	34.8	30	65.2	0	0.0

*Figures represent only reported assistance described as "very helpful" or "somewhat helpful."

†Percentages are noncumulative in that an individual may have reported more than one type of help from a given source. "Don't know," "not relevant," and insufficiently specific responses have been omitted.

≠Percentage not computed because of small N.

because of illness" may be important, the less severely ill also receive considerable support, aid, and services. An important differentiating variable may be social integration, as measured by level of social participation. The presence of nonreceivers of aid who are also possible social isolates points to a target group which may particularly require attention and assistance with their rehabilitation and adjustment to the illness.

SUMMARY

This chapter first reviewed patients' perceptions of some recent effects of their illness on other family members. About two-thirds of the married patients at Year 8 reported that their wives had been significantly affected. The response was most frequently expressed as anxiety and worry on the part of the wives. But relatively few of the women had changed life styles or roles in the family as a result of the illness. The perceived response to the illness by the wives and children at Year 8 differed by the level of severity of the man's illness. However, in general, wives were perceived as somewhat more affected than were the children. Few children had been limited in their social activities, education, or life plans by their fathers' illness. Only 14% of the married men reported at Year 8 that the illness had influenced their wives to maintain or seek employment. In the few families that were negatively affected by employment of the wives, the illness was not the major complicating factor.

In nearly one-third of the homes studied, at least one other family member had a significant illness or chronic health problem during the previous year. There was no apparent evidence, however, that the burden of illness in the home was triggered by stresses associated with the illness problems of the heart patient, and socioeconomic status was not associated with illness level in the home.

At Year 8 the health level of the patient was not associated with level of marital happiness. The most frequently mentioned area of disagreement between husbands and wives at Year 8 was the handling of family finances. Data suggested that the husband's illness level was inversely related to the presence of financial disagreement in the marriage. Forty percent of the "least severely ill" men reported some disagreement on finances, while only 11% of the "most ill" men cited finances as an area of disagreement.

Perceptions of protectiveness on the part of wives seemed to be unrelated to the severity of the husband's illness. Of those patients who responded that their wives were restrictive at Year 8, over four-fifths had responded affirmatively to the same question in interviews years earlier.

In rating important factors in the etiology of their illness, nearly one-fifth of all married patients at Year 8 cited conflicts with their wives and nearly one-fifth of fathers cited their children.

When sources of support and aid at Year 8 were examined,

both the extended kin group and quasi-kin appeared prominent. Children were a main source of aid in the form of services. The data showed a positive association between social integration as measured by social participation and receipt of aid. They suggest that the degree of social integration and not need in time of illness may determine who receives more support.

NOTES

1. "Major" illnesses were defined as those which were usually or possibly life-threatening. "Minor" illnesses were those which were usually not life-threatening and/or did not normally require operations or other medical treatment. Coding classification employed for the illness series was provided by Sol Levine and Norman A. Scotch from their study of social stress in the Framingham Heart Study population.

   Patients were asked whether any other family member in the household besides themselves had suffered from a serious illness or chronic health condition during the past year. Of the patients at Year 8, 67.8% responded that there was no other family member who had been ill. Thirty-one percent responded in the affirmative: 27.3% stated that one other person in their family had been sick, 3.4% named two family members and one patient (.5%) said that three persons in his household were seriously ill.

2. Only 8 patients had a parent living in their households at Year 8.

3. See also Croog and Levine (1977) for discussion of items and methods.

4. Definition and classification of "friends" and "neighbors" was not specified in the interview, but each respondent answered according to his own frame of reference. Obviously, there is some degree of overlap between the two categories.

5. Patients who responded that a category of kin or non-kin had been helpful were subsequently asked to specify the type of help provided. These were later coded in three classifications: "moral support," "services given," and "financial aid."

Chapter 7

PSYCHOLOGICAL CHARACTERISTICS AND EMOTIONAL STATUS OVER TIME

INTRODUCTION

In many ways personality mechanisms may constitute constructive means of coping with illness, serving as important means of defense or support in the "armory of resources." In managing their lives with illness, patients with high emotional stability, morale, and positive self-image have advantages over those who do not have these resources. In this chapter, employing empirical data from the 8-year study we can examine aspects of possible relationships between the illness experience and elements of personality.

Taking a longitudinal approach, this chapter considers areas relating to psychological characteristics and emotional status of men in the study population. These include: (1) stability and change in self-image over 8 years, as assessed through psychological self-rating items; (2) aspects of "cardiac personality" traits and the "coronary-prone behavior pattern"; (3) relationships between severity of illness and psychological characteristics; (4) depressive reaction and its correlates; and (5) subjective stress.

Our data on psychological characteristics reported in this

176

chapter are based in part on a set of 22 self-rating items, listed in Table 7-1. As we have noted earlier, at Week 7 patients were asked to rate themselves as they had been prior to the illness. At Year 1 and Year 8 they were asked to describe themselves on each item in regard to their current characteristics. At Year 1 wives were also asked to rate their husbands on the series of items. (See Note 1 for information on methods and on use of these and analogous items in research by others). In addition to these materials we draw upon patient responses to questions concerning their depressive reaction to the illness and concerning feelings of subjective stress.

Heart Disease and Self-Rated Psychological Characteristics: Year 8 and in Longitudinal Perspective

How patients perceive their own psychological characteristics bears on several important questions relevant to the conceptual and clinical issues of this book. The first concerns simply how patients with a chronic illness view themselves. A second issue concerns change and stability of psychological characteristics over time. This in turn relates to a larger matter central to studies of personality structure and process: the continuity of self-image over a period of years and the factors which may underlie stability and change.

As our interests are focused upon psychological characteristics in the context of a long-term disease, the analysis employs illness level as a principal independent variable. Thus, one of our prime concerns, for example, is whether the most severely ill men change more markedly than healthier patients in regard to emotional lability, depression, and such "coronary-risk" traits as aggressiveness, high ambition, and feeling pressed for time.

In addition to describing and documenting the characteristics of the heart patients over time, these materials may provide data relevant to other research on relationships between psychological characteristics and coronary heart disease. Theories concerning the possible relationship of personality type or psychological characteristics to heart disease have a long history, and in 1892 William Osler was among the first to suggest ways in

Table 7-1. Self-Rated Psychological Characteristics at Year 8.
Ranked by Percent of "High" Responses (N = 205)

Psychological Characteristic	Responses in Percent[*]		
	High	Medium	Low
Sense of duty	92.7	7.4	0
Puts a lot of effort into things	68.8	26.8	4.4
Sense of humor	66.4	33.6	0
Likes responsibility	64.9	28.8	6.3
Easygoing	59.5	34.7	5.9
Ambitious	47.8	37.5	14.6
Stubborn	38.5	55.1	6.3
Eats rapidly	36.6	30.3	32.7
In a hurry	29.8	43.9	26.3
Hard driving	26.9	36.1	37.1
Nervous	26.3	54.1	19.0
Feelings easily hurt	23.4	54.6	22.0
Easily angered	22.5	60.0	17.6
Easily excited	19.5	55.1	25.4
Likes organizations	18.1	36.1	44.4
Dominating or bossy	16.1	39.5	44.4
Critical of others	12.2	54.6	33.2
Moody	8.8	62.5	28.8
Shy	7.8	45.4	46.8
Self-centered	7.4	44.4	47.8
Easily depressed	7.3	46.8	45.4
Jealous	1.5	23.9	74.6

[*]High = very much or considerably; Medium = somewhat or a little;
Low = not at all. Percentages may not sum to 100 due to both rounding and the elimination of "no response" and "don't know" responses.

which the heart patient seemed distinctive in terms of personal traits. The main lines of clinical observations and empirical research in this area have been summarized many times, and two sets of reviews by Jenkins are among the most comprehensive (1971, 1976).

From research and clinical observations, some core themes concerning so-called "coronary personality" have emerged, and the characteristics reviewed in this chapter are similar to those which have often been used to describe the heart patient (Alexander, 1950; Dunbar, 1948; Jenkins, 1976). In some respects they also resemble characteristics commonly associated with the "Type A" personality or "coronary-prone behavior pattern" (Friedman & Rosenman, 1974). These, as summarized by Jenkins, are evident in "a style of behavior characterized by striving for achievement, competitiveness, impatience, time-urgency, dedication to a vocation or a profession, and excesses of drives and aggression" (1977).

These longitudinal materials were collected during a period when increasing research attention centered on the role of psychological and social characteristics as possible risk factors in the etiology of coronary disease and as elements affecting rehabilitation and recovery (Croog, 1978; Jenkins, 1976). The Type A coronary-prone behavior pattern, in particular, was given extended evaluation by panels of experts under the sponsorship of the National Heart, Lung, and Blood Institute (Dembroski, et al. 1978). While the evidence is not conclusive concerning the etiological role of psychological factors, some proponents maintain that it is now clear that heart patients are indeed distinctive in personal characteristics. For example, after a reassessment of a large series of data on myocardial infarction patients under age 65 in the Western Collaborative Group Study, Friedman recently remarked "I now believe that if we had known then what we now know about the detection of Type A behavior, almost every one of these men in 1960–61 would have been labelled Type A" (1979).

Our method of approaching the construct of a "coronary personality" cannot be considered as testing the validity of research findings and clinical observations in the scientific literature over past decades. Nor do our research results provide an assessment of the particular construct, Type A, or the "coronary-prone behavior pattern." One reason is that we used instruments different from those employed by other investigators. In regard to Type A, in particular, the construct is usually specified as that which is measured by the Standardized Interview of Friedman and Rosenman (1974) and the Jenkins Activity Scale (Jenkins, 1977). Individual items rather than scales were used in our study for the main analysis, and the effects of individual items are different from scales in terms of variance. However, we should note that for supplementary analysis we employed factor scores, derived from factor analysis based on the list of individual variables, to serve as composite indices.

As ours is not a direct test of the hypotheses on coronary disease and personality, we can only note some data and observations pertinent to the general issue as to whether there is a "coronary personality" as characterized over the decades since William Osler. Although our methods differ from other studies, we can nevertheless hypothesize that in a study population composed solely of middle-aged male heart patients, some relatively clear indications of "classic" traits should be prominent, such as ambition, aggressiveness, ease of anger, and time urgency.

Self-Rated Psychological Characteristics at Year 8

How do the patients in the study population view themselves at Year 8? A pattern of self-image, as revealed by ratings on individual psychological characteristics, is reported in Table 7-1.[1] The percentage distributions show that high proportions of the patients chose to characterize themselves as responsible and diligent persons. "Sense of duty," "putting effort into things," and "likes responsibility" are prominent ratings. A substantial minority, we can note, also characterized themselves as "high" in terms of ambition, being hard driving, eating rapidly, and being in a hurry.

Focus on these proportions should not obscure the fact of variation, however. On nearly all the items, patients ranged broadly in their responses. Hence, we must look beyond the picture of modal response and center on variation and its correlates. In our analysis, therefore, we examine the data with this theme in mind.

Factor Analysis and Psychological Characteristics of the Heart Patients

A factor analysis was performed to determine whether an underlying pattern of relationships existed within the set of psychological variables.[2] Seven principal factors emerged, with the first three accounting for 40% of the total variance (see Table 7–2). The first factor accounts for 19.6% of variance; we have termed it "emotional lability." The items with greatest loadings on this factor were "nervous," "easily excited," and "feelings easily hurt." The second factor, termed "dominance," accounts for 13% of the total variance. Items with highest loadings were "critical of others," "bossy," and "hard-driving." The third factor, labeled "ambition," explains 7% of the total variance. "Being ambitious," "likes responsibility," and "puts a lot of effort into things," had the greatest loadings.

Several features of the factor analysis are noteworthy. First, the same pattern of factors emerged from a factor analysis of these identical items from the cohorts at Week 7 and Year 1. The analysis is reported in our first book, *The Heart Patient Recovers* (1977). As we shall see, the similar results are indeed due in part

Table 7–2. Factor Analysis of Self-Rated Psychological Characteristics. Product at Year 8 (N = 198). Rotated Factor Loadings.

Factor 1: Emotional Lability (19.6%)[*]		Factor 2: Dominance (13.0%)	
Nervous	.757	Critical of others	.758
Easily excited	.650	Dominating or bossy	.577
Feelings easily hurt	.496	Hard driving	.485
Easily angered	.494	Stubborn	.371
Easily depressed	.491	Self-centered	.366
Moody	.402	Easily excited	.331

Factor 3: Ambition (7.0%)	
Ambitious	.809
Likes responsibility	.431
Puts effort into things	.418
Hard driving	.292

[*]The numbers in parentheses after each of the factors represent the percentage of variance accounted for by each factor.

to the high consistency of responses by individual patients over the years on these items.

Factor analysis assesses the underlying pattern of relationships in a set of variables, usually for purposes of data reduction. It does not describe the degree to which individual men can be characterized by the factors. It is interesting, nevertheless, that two of the factors we found, "ambition" and "dominance," are consistent with hypotheses of "coronary-prone behavior pattern."

Some perspective on the relative importance of the factors "ambition" and "dominance" can be gained from the fact that the two together account for only 20% of the variance, an amount equivalent to that of the single first factor, "emotional lability." Further, in evaluating these data, we must emphasize that on the individual items which make up the factors, high proportions of the heart patients did not characterize themselves as markedly ambitious, pressed for time, or as having other traits associated with Type A behavior pattern.

In sum, what do these distributions mean? As a whole, these findings on individual self-ratings indicate that in this population of heart patients many did not describe themselves as having characteristics commonly identified with classic descriptions of the coronary personality. These findings are similar to those which emerged in the heart patient population at an earlier stage in their illness careers—the period following their first myocardial infarction (Croog & Levine, 1977). Nevertheless, we must point out that theories of coronary personality or of behavior pattern hold that a particular individual need only be characterized by some, not by all, of a series of key traits (Dembroski et al., 1978). Hence, the distributions on individual characteristics reported here may not be inconsistent with current theories concerning personality pattern of the heart patient. However, future research making use of a control group could help explain whether these findings relate to the heart patients in particular or whether they are primarily characteristic of males in our American cultural context emphasizing drive, achievement, and ambition.

With this background, we now turn to several analytic issues involving psychological items and factor scores over the 8-year study period.

Illness Experience and Psychological Characteristics: A Longitudinal Approach

Illness and Changes in Self-Ratings. A first issue involves the possible influence of illness on psychological self-assessments in our study population. How stable were self-rated psychological characteristics of the heart patients? In which particular characteristics did they show the most change? Is change in self-image over a period of years associated with illness level?

To answer these questions, we compared patients' self-ratings of pre-illness and Year 1 characteristics with those at Year 8. The first rating, we should recall, was made 1 month after return home from the hospital and thus was a retrospective assessment. The Year 1 ratings were self-assessments at the current time.

In our base-line study (Croog & Levine, 1977), we found a high association between ratings on pre-illness psychological items and Year 1. The prospect of examining stability and change in responses to the same items after 8 years thus was an intriguing one.

Statistically, responses remained relatively stable for pre-illness, Year 1 and Year 8 (see Table 7-3). Comparing pre-illness ratings with those at Year 8 for each man, gamma scores ranged from .37 to .77. The most stability in gamma scores appears in such items as "eats rapidly," "likes organizations," and "sense of duty." Those responses which changed the most were "easily excited," "hard-driving," and "dominating or bossy."

For most of the items in which there was change, there was little difference between the total percentage moving upward and the total percentage moving downward. Over the long term, notable percentage net change in a single direction occurred on only 4 items in the list of 22 (column D). These were "in a hurry," "hard-driving," and "ambitious," and "eats rapidly." Among these items, the net change downward was relatively substantial for only one: 21% in the case of "in a hurry." On the whole, however, there may be suggestive signs in these data among men with characteristics commonly associated with "coronary personality," there was no substantial change downward in the series of main items, and chance may account for the minor variation.

As might be expected, a pattern of stability similar to that for

Table 7-3. Stability of Self-Rated Psychological Characteristics
From Week 7 Assessments of Pre-Illness Status to Year 8.
Base N = 205

Psychological Characteristic*	Gamma Score	A Percent of Patients Reporting Stability in Item	B Percent of Patients Reporting Increase in Item	C Percent of Patients Reporting Decrease in Item	D Net Difference (B - C)
Eats rapidly	.77	62.7	13.3	24.0	-10.7
Likes organizations	.72	59.4	19.3	21.3	- 2.0
Sense of duty	.68	85.8	9.8	4.4	5.4
Sense of humor	.67	69.3	16.6	14.1	2.5
Shy	.67	60.9	16.6	22.5	- 5.9
Ambitious	.66	59.5	14.7	25.8	-11.1
Puts effort into things	.64	71.7	9.3	19.1	- 9.8
Easygoing	.62	61.5	15.1	23.4	- 8.3
Feelings easily hurt	.62	56.5	25.0	18.6	6.4
In a hurry	.61	50.8	14.1	35.1	-21.0
Nervous	.60	53.2	25.2	21.7	3.5
Critical of others	.60	58.5	21.4	20.0	1.4
Easily depressed	.60	59.5	19.3	21.2	- 1.9

Table 7-3 (Continued)

Psychological Characteristic	Gamma Score	A Percent of Patients Reporting Stability in Item	B Percent of Patients Reporting Increase in Item	C Percent of Patients Reporting Decrease in Item	D Net Difference (B − C)
Jealous	.59	71.1	14.2	14.8	− .6
Likes responsibility	.59	63.4	21.0	15.6	5.4
Moody	.57	56.3	25.0	18.6	6.4
Self-centered	.55	57.7	21.7	20.7	1.0
Easily angered	.54	53.0	24.0	23.1	.9
Stubborn	.52	57.4	22.1	20.6	1.5
Dominating or bossy	.47	48.1	28.0	24.0	4.0
Hard driving	.41	48.8	18.6	32.7	−14.1
Easily excited	.37	49.4	26.0	24.5	1.5

*For purposes of this table, the five original response categories were condensed to three: High, Medium, and Low. Column A includes respondents in all three categories whose rating remained stable. Percentages do not sum to 100 in all cases due to rounding.

the pre-illness-Year 8 comparison also characterized the comparison of the Year 1-Year 8 time points.

Results from these data on the population as a whole are mirrored when we consider only those men who have a potential for change in a particular direction. For example, among those men who are classified in the "high" category on our scale, the only possible change is downward, and conversely, among those men already in the "low" category, the only possible direction for change is upward. In a separate analysis, we therefore selected out those men in the high and medium categories in order to examine patterns of stability and of change downward. Using the same method, we combined men in the low and medium categories to examine stability and possible change upward. These procedures were also followed in our earlier report on the first year after the heart attack (1977).

As in the case of the first-year data, no consistent pattern emerged indicating a change in self-perception over time on key items relating to classic "coronary personality" descriptors. In other words, with the passage of 8 years and the inevitable processes associated with aging, the proportions reporting increase in aggressiveness, ambition, and emotional lability were on the whole similar to those reporting decrease.

Was long-term change in psychological self-ratings related to severity of cardiac illness? To explore this matter, ratings on each pre-illness item were compared with scores at Year 8, controlling for cardiac illness level by using rehospitalization history. Three groups were compared: (1) those never rehospitalized for heart disease; (2) those rehospitalized once; and (3) those rehospitalized two or more times.

The pattern of stability and change did not differ significantly among the three groups. Similar results emerged from the comparison of Year 1 and Year 8 data as measured by partial gamma scores. Further analysis employing physician ratings of impairment as a measure of illness level at Year 1 and Year 8 also produced nonsignificant differences. In other words, when these comparisons were made we did not find that changes in self-ratings from one time point to another were related to illness level.

Illness and Current Self-Ratings.   A related question is whether severity of illness at Year 8 is related to concurrent psychological self-ratings. A corollary question at Year 8 is whether those men most heavily burdened with heart disease are those most characterized by descriptors associated with the "coronary personality." For example, were those men who were currently the most ambitious and time pressured also the most ill; or, in other words, was the level of current ambition or of feeling time pressure associated with illness level?

For economy of effort, the analysis was first pursued through use of the Year 8 factor scores we discussed earlier. The score of each individual on each of the three factors was specified. A series of t tests were then carried out comparing the mean "emotional lability," "dominance" and "ambition" factor scores for pairs of groups with differing illness histories. The groups were: (1) not rehospitalized for any reason since Week 7; (2) rehospitalized once for heart-related reasons; and (3) rehospitalized for heart disease two or more times since Week 7.[3]

No significant differences were found between men in different illness level categories with regard to scores on "dominance" and "ambition." With regard to "emotional lability," however, there were significant differences between the mean factor scores and the two extreme groups: "not rehospitalized" and those "rehospitalized twice or more." Mean scores on the factor were .34 for the "two or more rehospitalizations" group and −.09 for the nonrehospitalized men (t = 2.70, d.f. = 46.9, $p < .05$).[4] This finding thus suggests only that patients with the most rehospitalizations for heart disease were more emotionally labile than nonrehospitalized men.

We next examined scores on *individual* psychological items in the factors at Year 8, comparing pairs of the illness level groups, in order to discern differences in pattern which might have been obscured by the factor analysis method. On the whole, the results of t tests on individual items do not differ from the results based on the factor scores. For example, on those individual items comprising the "emotional lability" factor, such as "nervous," "angers easily," and "feelings easily hurt," the two extreme illness level groups also differed significantly. The intermediate illness severity group did not differ from either of the other two groups on any items.

In other words, on both the individual items and the factor

scores for "dominance" and "ambition" the most severely ill men at Year 8 exhibited the same psychological characteristics as the healthier men. The relationship between severity of illness and "emotional lability" at Year 8 deserves special note. An obvious interpretation, of course, is that multiple hospitalizations are associated with higher emotional stress. We can be tempted to conclude that these data describe only a reactive emotional state, stemming from the prospect that the most severely ill men at Year 8 simply have more to worry about. Hence, those men who have the most uncertain future and who are burdened with additional illness, are the most nervous, easily excited, and easily angered, as indicated by these data. However, the role of emotional factors in the complex illness processes leading to the rehospitalizations cannot be discounted. The "emotional lability" factor may be associated with a tendency toward subsequent cardiac events, and its etiological role deserves further scrutiny. Other hypotheses and explanations deserve future exploration as well.

Year 1 to Year 8: Did Attrition Because of Heart Attacks in Men with Particular Psychological Characteristics Lead to the Year 8 Results?

In line with our goal to describe illness levels at Year 8 and psychological characteristics, we have centered thus far primarily on concurrent phenomena. A key question concerns whether the general lack of relationship between illness level and psychological characteristics at Year 8 can be explained by an attrition factor over the years. For example, are these results in some way due to the possibility that patients with particularly strong ambition, time urgency, or dominance had fatal heart attacks during the 7 years after Year 1 and thus were removed from the study?

We have already answered this question in Chapter 2, although from a somewhat different perspective. There we were concerned with the relationship between psychological characteristics pre-illness and at Year 1 as predictors of later health status. As the matter is relevant here as well, some brief recapitulation of the findings and background data may be useful.

As we pointed out in Chapter 2, the 22 psychological rating items examined individually were not related to subsequent coronary deaths. Further examination of the items through factor analysis at Year 1 showed no significant association with coronary deaths as of Year 8. Hence, we cannot conclude that the findings at Year 8 were due to the screening out of men who had particularly strong coronary-risk characteristics as shown on the earlier ratings. This is also another way of saying that over the 8-year period high ratings on the so-called "coronary-type" psychological items were not useful predictors of later coronary mortality.

Wives of the Heart Patients After 8 Years: A Research Note

In our base-line study (1977) we interviewed the wives of the heart patients, using an interview format similar in many respects to that employed for the patients themselves. We collected data on self-ratings of psychological characteristics concerning pre-illness and Year 1 periods, using the same 22 item series as we had for the men. We have reported elsewhere (Croog, Koslowsky, & Levine, 1976) that in those ratings similar percentages of the husband population and the wife population had such characteristics as ambition, time urgency, and other descriptors commonly cited by researchers on psychosocial factors in coronary disease.[5] Another feature of these data was that in husband-wife pairs, strong associations appeared between one spouse's self-ratings and the independent assessment of that spouse by the other. In the typical case, for example, the husband agreed independently with the wife's ratings of her own characteristics.

The particular matter of note here is that at the time of the base-line study, one male heart patient population and one nonheart patient group of wives did not differ in the patterning of psychological self-rated characteristics. Various explanations for the finding could be offered. One is that particular characteristics rated as "coronary prone" are male sex-typed, and are not prominent in women in this age group. Another is that the women with such characteristics are perhaps really a latent heart patient population. As heart disease develops more slowly in women than in men during the middle years, perhaps they were fated to have later manifestations of the acute phase.

Psychological characteristics of women in relation to heart disease have only relatively rarely been examined (Bengtsson, Hallstrom, & Tibblin, 1973; Haynes & Feinleib, 1980; Kenigsberg et al., 1974; Rosenman & Friedman, 1961; Shekelle, Schoenberger, & Stamler, 1976). Hence, at least a brief note of the subsequent fate of the wives after 8 years perhaps deserves mention here.

Ninety-five percent of the men married at Year 8 were still wed to the same women as at the time of the first interview. The wives were on the average 2 years younger than the husbands, and their mean age at Year 8 was 57. Although they were entering the age period of increased risk of heart disease, we would expect to find in this age group rates equal to a fraction of that in the general male population (Bengtsson, Hallstrom, & Tibblin, 1973; Kannel, Sorlie, & McNamara, 1979).

It was not possible to interview the wives of the heart patients in connection with the Year 8 study. However, through reports by the husbands participating at Year 8, some information on the illness history of the wives is available, covering the period from Year 1 to Year 8.

Only 13 men reported at Year 8 that their wives were ill with either a chronic or acute condition involving disease of the cardiovascular system. There were four men whose wives had died between Week 7 and Year 8. Even if we assume that all four women died of heart disease, this would mean that in the select population of 175 surviving married or widowed male heart patients at Year 8, about 10% ($N = 17$) had wives with heart disease, according to these data and assumptions.

Thus, while approximately 75% of the male heart patient group suffered death or rehospitalization for heart disease over the course of 8 years, the wife population remained comparatively well in terms of cardiac health. The small number of cardiac events among the wives over the 8 years precludes meaningful analysis of their earlier psychological self-ratings in relation to their cardiac mortality and morbidity. However, as we noted, the wives' self-ratings as a group were similar to the patterning for a male heart patient group—their husbands. Such data help point up the possibility that, should psychological characteristics constitute significant risk factors in coronary disease, their complex functioning may be very different in the two sexes.[6]

HEART DISEASE AND DEPRESSIVE REACTION

In the literature on the role of emotions in etiology of illness, there is a continuing debate concerning depression as a precipitating factor, and as a complication affecting recovery and rehabilitation (Basch, 1975; Becker, 1974; Bibring, 1953; Engel & Ader, 1967). In heart disease, as in many other chronic illnesses, one of the main emotional problems is depression. Since many heart patients are depressed, questions persist as to whether they are depressed mainly as a consequence of heart disease, or whether their heart disease is in some way a consequence of their depression. Indeed, the depression often may be clearly associated with the illness as a reactive response. Because he has heart disease, a patient may become depressed as he recognizes the long-term debilitating, disabling, and possibly lethal consequences of the illness. Or the depression may be primarily endogenous, characteristic of the individual. Some of the other sources of the depression may be biochemical, either naturally occurring neurohumeral responses, or side-effects induced by drugs employed in the medical regimen.

Problems of research on depression are often complicated by issues of conceptualization and measurement. In a technical sense the phenomenon is, after all, a construct, one which "exists" by virtue of the fact that it is conceived, labeled, and measured. Depression can be viewed as a mood, symptom, or syndrome, and much controversy exists in regard to issues of validity, reliability, or replicability in depression studies (Fieve, 1971; Kendell, 1977; Weissman & Paykel, 1974).

Depressive reaction as a complicating factor in many chronic illnesses has been relatively neglected, compared with the rich effusion of research on depression in psychiatric patients. But the complex relationship between depression and heart disease in particular has increasingly drawn the attention of researchers in recent years. The data from our heart patient population have offered us prospects for exploring the depressive phenomenon in a sizeable group of men from a prospective viewpoint.

Depressive Reaction and Its Correlates: Aspects of Construct Validity

Our primary concern here is with one aspect of the larger phenomenon of "depression"—*depressive reaction to heart disease.*[7] At Year 1 and Year 8 patients were asked a series of questions bearing on mood and their response to the illness. Among the intercorrelated measures, we have selected the patient's report of being depressed as our primary item for this analysis. Thus, at both Year 1 and Year 8 patients were labeled as having reported "depressive reaction" if they answered affirmatively when asked, "Do you ever feel discouraged or depressed over your illness."[8] Follow-up questions then focused on the frequency and intensity of depressive reaction at that time as well.

Some clues about the validity of our measures of the depressive reaction construct are furnished by an examination of correlates. In addition to its face validity, our main measure is correlated with characteristics consistent with reported depressive reaction. As Table 7-4 shows, the depressive reaction response at Year 1 and/or Year 8 was related to a series of items, showing positive associations with subjective stress, bodily complaints, and a negative view of the progress of recovery. It was negatively associated with quality of life measures, such as life satisfaction, finding positive meaning in the illness, and feelings of achievement of personal goals (Croog & La Voie, 1980).

Given the interview context and the social implications of depressive reaction, we assume that the factor of social acceptability was an element influencing responses of patients. Unquestionably some men with depressive reaction preferred not to reveal their feelings of despair over the illness. Hence, the actual prevalence is larger in some degree than the percentages reported. Rather than center upon prevalence, our primary focus here is, therefore, upon the correlates of given responses over time within our study group, using a panel approach.

Depressive Reaction at Year 1 and Year 8.

Let us first examine reported depressive reaction earlier in the illness in relation to its later occurrence at Year 8. Patients

Table 7-4. Relationship Between Reported Depressive Reaction and Other
           Variables. Gamma Scores at Year 1 and Year 8 and
           Level of Significance on Chi-Square Test

| | Reported Depressive Reaction | | | |
| | Year 1 (N = 293) | | Year 8 (N = 205) | |
Variable	Gamma	p	Gamma	p
Life Returned to Normal	-.81	.01	*	-
Number of Symptoms	.66	.01	.52	.01
Patient's View of His Progress	-.53	.01	*	-
Satisfaction With Life	-.39	.01	-.67	.01
Maintenance of Pre-Illness Activity Level	-.34	.01	*	-
Perceived Gains from the Illness	-	NS	-.57	.01
Subjective Stress Scale	≠	-	.48	.01
Positive Change in Attitude Toward Life	-	NS	-.38	.01
Achievement of Life Goals	-.40	.01	-.38	.01

*Item was not included in Year 8 interviews.

≠The full Subjective Stress Scale was not included in Year 1 interviews.

NS = not significant.

were first directly questioned about depressive reaction at Year 1.
As Table 7-5 shows, the positive response on depressive reaction
at that time was significantly associated with the same response 7
years later. Further, controlling for level of illness at Year 1, those
who were "most ill" and who were depressed were most likely to
report depressive reaction 7 years later as well.

At this point, it is useful to recall some earlier findings on
outcomes after Year 1. As we noted in Chapter 2, reported
depressive reaction at Year 1 was associated with significantly
higher risk of death from heart disease over the follow-up period.
This would be expected on the basis of the association between
depressive reaction and the illness stimulus itself: men with severe cardiac disease were also more likely to be depressed, and

Table 7-5.   Depressive Reaction at Year 8 by Depressive Reaction at
             Year 1.   Total Participants and by Illness Level.

	Depressive Reaction at Year 1	Depressive Reaction at Year 8		
		Yes Percent (N)	No Percent (N)	Total N
Total Participants at Year 8	Yes	34.7 (33)	65.3 (62)	100.0 (95)
	No	14.8 (16)	85.2 (92)	100.0 (108)
	Total N	49	154	203*

Chi-square = 9.87, d.f. = 1, p<.01

By Physician's Rating of Patient's Functional Health Status at Year 1[†]

a) No Significant Impairment	Yes	26.8 (11)	73.2 (30)	100.0 (41)
	No	13.6 (9)	86.4 (57)	100.0 (66)
	Total N	20	87	107

Chi-square = 2.09, d.f. = 1, p<.20

b) Moderate or Severe Impairment	Yes	43.9 (18)	56.1 (23)	100.0 (41)
	No	16.0 (4)	84.0 (21)	100.0 (25)
	Total N	22	44	66

Chi-square = 4.26, d.f. = 1, p<.05

*"No response" has been omitted.

[†]Physicians' ratings were unavailable for some patients.   See Note 2, Chapter 2.

many died. Hence, the removal from the study population of those patients most severely affected modifies the differences at Year 8 shown in Table 7-5. Nonetheless, the higher risk for subsequent depressive reaction at Year 8 is still evident among those survivors who had reported depressive reaction at Year 1.

Association between concurrent depressive reaction and severity of illness at Year 1 was also matched in the Year 8 data. For example, of those who were most ill at Year 8 as rated by their physicians, 46% reported depressive reaction at that time; of those who were rated least impaired, only 18% did so (chi-square = 9.507, d.f. = 2, $p < .01$, gamma = .48).

These data imply that at an early stage after myocardial infarction, it may be possible to assess relative risk of depressive reaction years later on the basis of severity of cardiac illness and concurrent depressive reaction.

Predisposition to Depression and Depressive Reaction.

Depressive reaction associated with heart disease clearly has different implications for patients with high predisposition to depression than for those who were rarely, if ever, depressed before the heart attack (Kendell, 1977). In the case of our study group, do subsequent health careers differ when we compare (1) men with reported marked tendencies for depression and (2) men with minimal depressive tendencies? Our data collected on reported susceptibility to depression before and after the illness, as well as our data on depressive reaction, allow exploration of the question and some related matters.

As Table 7-1 shows, being "easily depressed" was among the 22 self-rated psychological items. As we have explained earlier, the ratings on this and other characteristics were made in regard to pre-illness status, Year 1 and Year 8. Distributions of the ratings were earlier discussed as well.

Indications of construct validity of the "easily depressed" item are furnished by the pattern of its correlates. In the pre-illness period, for example, reported ratings show it was significantly associated with such other pre-illness items as moodiness, nervousness, ease of anger, and other measures of emotional reactivity. Further, as we have reported earlier (Croog, Koslowsky & Levine, 1977), there is some notable consistency between ways in which married patients viewed themselves and their wive's assessment of them. In both the pre-illness and the Year 1 ratings, there was significant association between the patient's self assessment and his wife's ratings of his being "easily depressed." Agreement between husband and wife in regard to the patient's emotional state is not a systematic measure, of course, but in conjunction with the other evidence cited, it constitutes a consensual support for the validity of the item.

One feature of these data is the continuity and stability of the "easily depressed" responses from one time point to another. Among those core 205 men who participated in all four interview stages of the study, the gamma correlation between pre-illness "easily depressed" and the Year 8 rating is .60; between Year 1 and Year 8 it is .45. Similar stability characterized responses of the total study group between adjacent time points.

Being seriously ill did not appear to be related to the "easily depressed" response. At both Year 1 and Year 8 rehospitalization history was employed as a measure of illness level to determine whether being currently "easily depressed" varied as a function of severity of illness. No significant differences were found. Similar lack of association emerged when we employed our other measures of illness level as well. Further, as we pointed out in Chapter 2, being "easily depressed" at Year 1 did not have predictive value in assessing risk for later negative health status. Like the other psychological items in the 22-item series, "easily depressed" at Year 1 was not related to subsequent mortality or cardiovascular morbidity, as measured at Year 8.

The relationship between being "easily depressed" pre-illness and later depressive reaction to the illness presents a mixed picture. We found a relationship between (1) the rating of pre-illness tendency toward depression, and (2) reported illness-related depressive reaction at 1 year (gamma = .36, chi-square = 13.64, d.f. = 2, $p < .001$). In other words, those describing themselves as easily depressed before the illness were most likely to report depressive reaction 1 year after the initial acute episode. However, this significant relationship was not maintained when the "pre-illness" rating on "easily depressed" was examined in relation to the illness-related depressive reaction at Year 8.

These data suggest that depressive reaction at Year 1 was influenced by a predisposition to depression before the first heart attack. But being "easily depressed" before the illness had limited utility in predicting possible risk of depressive reaction at 8 years.

Subjective Stress, Depressive Reaction, and Correlates

Among many patients, reports of depressive reaction to the illness were accompanied by reports of anxiety, tension, or stress.

This constellation of emotions constitutes a common clinical picture, and it is not surprising that it is reflected in our data as well. For example, patients' reports of depressive reaction at Year 8 were positively associated with scores at that time on the "emotional lability" factor. The psychological items with the highest loadings on this factor were "nervous," "feelings easily hurt," and "easily excited," all of which may indicate intense emotional response to stress.

Other assessments of nervousness, tension, and emotional strain in the study population at Year 8 were derived from scores on the Subjective Stress Scale developed by Reeder and colleagues (Reeder et al., 1973). Patients were asked to specify the degree to which a series of four statements described them in regard to current feelings of being under stress. Scores for all patients were then grouped into terciles designating subjective stress as "high," "medium," and "low."[9]

The positive association between reports of depressive reaction and subjective stress at Year 8 is relatively clear (see Table 7-4). Of those patients who stated at Year 8 that they were depressed because of their illness, 40% reported "high" stress in terms of the scale items, and 17% reported "low" stress. In contrast, of those who reported no depressive reaction, 45% were in the "low" stress group, while only 21% characterized themselves as "highly" stressed (chi-square $= 13.89$, d.f. $= 2$, $p < .001$, gamma $= .48$).

These findings on the total study group reaffirm a consistent picture of relationship between our measures of subjective stress and depressive reaction. However, whether the level of subjective stress is a function of other independent variables requires answers to a set of related questions. For example, is level of subjective stress at Year 8 related to the degree of impairment or health status? Does level of stress vary between subgroups with differing social or situational characteristics?

First, we turn to the issue of illness level and subjective stress at Year 8. Are the most ill men those who report the greatest subjective stress? We found no association between subjective stress level at Year 8 and health measures, such as the physicians' ratings of patients in regard to functional capacity and impairment. Second, data on the patients at Year 8 reveal no consistent, linear relationship between scores of the Subjective Stress Scale and such demographic and socioeconomic characteristics as age, educational level, occupational level, and income.

As might be expected, significant negative relationships were found between level of subjective stress at Year 8 and some indicators of social support and positive morale among the patients. These include such variables as: (1) marital happiness; (2) presence of a confidant; (3) report of life satisfaction; and (4) feeling of achievement of life goals. Conversely, there were statistically significant positive relationships between subjective stress level and (1) reported marital disagreement; (2) high scores on the "emotional lability" factor; (3) stress and tension at work; and (4) job dissatisfaction.

In sum, illness level at Year 8 and demographic and socioeconomic characteristics of patients did not appear to be useful as possible "predictors" of their level of reported subjective stress. Instead, such reported stress appeared to be part of a larger picture of dysphoria.

These findings based on patients' reports are consistent in many ways with reports of subjective stress by their wives. (Croog & Fitzgerald, 1978.) Our earlier study of the wives suggested also that level of subjective stress was one aspect of a more general stress experience, expressed also in emotional lability and feelings of unhappiness in marriage. Their reported stress level was not a simple correlate of such variables as severity of illness of the husband, burden of illness in the home, age of the wife, or socioeconomic status.

We will also consider subjective stress in Chapter 8, where we focus on antecedents and correlates of "outcome" variables at Year 8.

SUMMARY

This chapter examined five areas relating to longitudinal patterning of psychological characteristics and heart disease: (1) psychological self-ratings of the study group over 8 years; (2) issues of the "coronary personality"; (3) illness level and changes in psychological characteristics; (4) depressive reaction and its correlates; and (5) relationships between depressive reaction and subjective stress. We examined psychological traits and states by means of a series of 22 self-rating items. Through factor analysis, we reduced the 22 items to three clusters of related variables labeling these "emotional lability," "dominance," and "ambition."

Patterns of psychological characteristics in the men at Year 8 were essentially similar to those prior to the illness and at Year 1, suggesting a high degree of consistency throughout the study period.

Stability and change in psychological self-ratings over the study period did not appear to be related to severity of illness in this patient population. Further, those with the most serious cardiac status at Year 8 did not differ from the less ill in psychological characteristics often associated with the "coronary-prone" personality. However, at the time of Year 8, men who had been rehospitalized for heart-related reasons had higher scores on the "emotional lability" factor at Year 8 than those not rehospitalized. This might be mainly a reactive phenomenon, in that those patients who suffered the most were perhaps those with most cause to be nervous, easily angered, and excited.

In this population of heart patients, a large segment did not describe themselves as having characteristics commonly associated with "coronary personality" or with "Type A" behavior pattern. This was consistent with findings of our baseline study, *The Heart Patient Recovers.*

At Year 8 positive associations between depressive reaction and (1) subjective stress and (2) bodily complaints were found. As might be expected, a negative association emerged between depressive reaction and ratings of quality of life. Indicators of depressive reaction to the illness at Year 1 were associated with indicators of depressive reaction at Year 8 as well. However, the characteristic, "easily depressed," rated early in the illness was not subsequently related statistically to depressive reaction at Year 8. At both Year 1 and Year 8 the reported depressive reaction was associated with concurrent severity of illness measures.

Patients' scores on both the "emotional lability" factor and the Subjective Stress Scale were positively related to depressive reaction to the illness. No relationships emerged between subjective stress and (1) severity of illness at Year 8 and (2) selected socioeconomic and demographic variables. We suggested that stress responses seemed to be a part of a more general pattern of affective responses, such as marital unhappiness, emotional lability, job dissatisfaction, and work stress.

Notes

1. For information on analyses based on similar items, see the articles by Haynes and colleagues (1978, 1980) based on the Framingham Heart Study population.

    The materials reported are based upon a series of 22 self-rating items descriptive of psychological characteristics. The series was derived from two sources. Seventeen items were employed in scales by Burgess and Wallin for marital prediction studies (1953). In addition, a series of five items was added by the authors. These were drawn from current conceptions about common components in the coronary personality, and they deal with such dimensions as feeling time pressure, being hard driving, and the exerting of effort. Patients were asked to rate themselves on each item using a five-point scale ranging from "very much" to "not at all." For some purposes, such as Table 7-1, the initial five categories were condensed. The responses "very much" and "considerably" were combined and coded as 1. The categories "somewhat" and "a little" were classified as a single category and were given a code rating of 2. Category 3 consisted of those responses which were "hasn't the characteristic at all."

2. Factor analysis was carried out through the use of the SPSS Program on the Univac 1106. The standard principal components factor analysis was computed for the total cohort at Year 8 of 205 respondents and for 22 individual items. The criteria for extracting roots were as follows: maximum number of factors = 8.0. Minimum latent root = 1.00. The minimum percent of communality was set at 10.00. Rotation of the seven factors which emerged was carried out through the Orthogonal Varimax technique. Each psychological variable was run with its original five coding categories.

3. Men rehospitalized for nonheart reasons were excluded in order to enable assessment of psychological items specifically in relation to

heart disease. However, separate analysis shows that even inclusion of this group does not alter the results reported here.

4. The separate variance-estimate method was used in this case since a preliminary F test indicated unequal sample variances. Hence, d.f. = 46.9 rather than 106.

5. This similarity cannot be explained as a "like marries like" phenomenon, since gamma scores comparing husband and wife self-ratings were small.

6. For findings on psychosocial characteristics as risk factors in coronary heart disease among women in Framingham, Massachusetts, see Haynes and colleagues (1978, 1980). As noted, the reports are based on psychosocial scales, constructed in part with items similar or analogous to those used in this study and our earlier baseline report (1977).

7. In the discussion of depressive reaction to heart disease in this book, it should be clear that we are referring to a phenomenon other than the psychiatric diagnostic syndrome, "reactive depression," as defined in the *Diagnostic and Statistical Manual* of the American Psychiatric Association.

8. In our first book, *The Heart Patient Recovers* (1977), we referred to feelings of depression or discouragement to designate responses to this question.

9. Patients were asked to specify the degree to which each of the following statements described them: (1) "At the end of the day I am completely exhausted mentally and physically"; (2) "There is a great amount of nervous strain connected with my daily activities"; (3) "My daily activities are extremely trying and stressful"; and (4) "In general I am unusually tense and nervous." The four possible responses to each statement were weighted as follows: "very well," 1 point; "fairly well," 2 points; "not very well," 3 points; "not at all," 4 points. A patient's total score on the 16-point index was the sum of his scores on each individual question. Responses were coded in terciles as follows: 15, 16 = "low" stress; 11–14 = "moderate" stress; 10 and under = "high" stress.

Chapter 8

THE PATIENT AFTER EIGHT YEARS

Factors Associated with Differing Patterns of Life Adjustment

After 8 years, how were the patients doing? How had their heart disease influenced the quality of their lives? What was the nature of their personal adaptation to the illness? Could patient characteristics previously identified in the base-line study have been used to predict how they would fare at Year 8? Beyond these questions concerning long-term predictors and descriptors, we have a primary concern with ways in which various elements in the "armory of resources" relate to the health of patients and their social and psychological adjustments at the end of 8 years.

In this chapter we pursue our inquiry through (1) focusing upon resources from the earlier base-line period and their relation to outcome 7 or 8 years later, and (2) examining resources in the current situations of patients in relation to their health, social, and emotional statuses.

In the next page, we outline two major facets of our approach: (1) conceptualization of Year 8 outcomes in terms of a series of status variables, and (2) the operational use of the "armory of resources" as a means of examining their role as antecedents and current correlates of outcome. Readers with only a secondary interest in methodological details and analytic

202

procedures may wish to turn directly to the findings reported in the latter portion of this chapter.

Approaches to "Outcome:" Multiple Status Measures

Primary and Secondary Status Variables at Year 8.   Our first consideration of "outcome' in Chapter 2 centered on the issues of death and survival in the study population. Subsequent chapters have focused solely upon the survivors, primarily upon their characteristics and circumstances in individual major areas of their lives and activities. In this chapter we turn to a more comprehensive or global assessment of outcomes at Year 8.

In longitudinal studies of patient populations, the situation of the patients relative to their illnesses has often been approached through measures of "adaptation" or "adjustment." In this report we examine outcome through conceptualizing the total situation of a patient at a particular point in time as consisting of a series of "statuses." These statuses are visualized in relation to major life areas, such as those reviewed in this report: work, family, interpersonal relationships, physical health, emotional health, and personal view of life. Within each area, patient statuses are then assessed in terms of a limited series of categories, and the rating indicates his position or rank on the status item. In the case of cardiac symptoms, for example, the relevant status scale possibilities might be "currently reports chest pain," and "currently does not report chest pain." In the case of a mental health item: "depressed" or "not depressed" are possible examples.

We use the status measure items simply as means of describing the study population, and an individual item, as employed here, has no implicit favorable or pejorative implication. In some cases, for example, being currently employed may be a highly favorable trait. In other circumstances, the descriptor, currently employed, may refer to highly undesirable circumstances, particularly for patients in health-endangering occupations.

Our purpose, therefore, is to avoid classifying individuals in relation to some hypothetical standard of adjustment, or "good health." Instead, we shall describe the various statuses of patients at particular points in time. Our emphasis first is upon which segments of the population are in which particular categories or statuses. The same data can then be interpreted in terms of alternate frames of reference or alternate sets of values.

Although the individual status measures may be drawn from differing dimensions (health, family, work, interpersonal relationships, etc.), they are in many instances significantly related to one another. This is to be expected. A physically healthy man in our society is also likely to exhibit social and psychological characteristics commonly associated with health, in such areas as employment and social participation. We therefore could carry out a reductionist effort, inspecting the pattern of association between outcome variables, then selecting one or a few measures as representative of the whole. In fact, on a purely statistical basis we could determine whether a single variable or measure effectively summarizes all the others.

We have chosen to proceed along a different route. We have preferred to review a constellation of measures of some principal life areas of the patients. As we have noted, one of our primary aims is descriptive analysis of the study population. A related goal is to identify particular subsegments of the study group as target populations for the attention of health care practitioners, medical care planners, and public health administrators. Hence, as our purpose is descriptive, it has seemed important to report on each major sphere separately. Through these procedures we attempt to portray conditions and problems in the many relevant areas of life of the heart patients.

In some ways our analysis of statuses at Year 8 supplements and occasionally overlaps our earlier discussion of life areas. Although a few of the same variables are employed as in previous chapters, the analysis here differs in that it is concerned with systematic overview of a profile of key outcomes and of their possible antecedents. Thus, our profile measures center on the patients' capacity of functioning physically and socially, the inroads of illness upon their work capacity, their physical status, their emotional health, and their own views of the quality of life and the long-term meanings of their lives. Naturally, none of the measures can in any sense tap the full range of meanings and complexities in each of these areas in the lives of the patients. They are employed as limited operational measures for use in our exploratory examination of the life careers and experience of the heart patients.

Goals of Status Indices.   The status measures are classified into two principal categories: primary and secondary.

Three primary status variables are devised as a triangulation on the condition of the patient at Year 8. They are based upon (1) criteria drawn from the world of work: employment status; (2) the clinical judgment of the physician; and (3) the patient's assessment of his own life situation. They center on three key aspects: work status, health, and quality of life.

The secondary status variables supplement the primary indices. They all draw on patients' reported perceptions and are concerned mainly with their views of their world, feelings about the meaning of their lives and achievements, and emotional states of depressive reaction, anxiety, and tension.

I.   The *primary status index variables* are as follows:

1. *Work and Retirement Status.* Two separate measures are employed. The first classifies the total study population in regard to the impact of illness on current work or retirement status. The second measure is concerned with current participation in the work force by nonretired men only.

Work-Retirement Status A. This variable distinguishes two categories of men: those who proceeded through the study period with "normal" work careers and those whose work careers were terminated or currently blocked by illness. The *first* category includes men of two types: (a) those in the work force at Year 8, or (b) those who retired for reasons not associated with illness. The *second* category consists of men whose work careers *were* illness affected: (a) they had been forced to retire by illness, or (b) they were currently unemployed because of illness.

We have called this category "illness-affected work career."

Current Work Status B. This measure pertains only to men who are nonretired and "work-force eligible." They are classified as either currently employed or currently unemployed at Year 8.

2. *Health Status: Physician Rating.* This item employs the physicians' ratings of functional health status, as used earlier in Chapter 2. The ratings range from "no significant impairment" to "severe impairment" or definite limitations on work and other activities.

3. *Satisfaction with Life: Report by Patient.* This item is based on the patient's self-assessment in response to the question, "On the whole, how satisfied are you with your life today?"

II. *The secondary status index variables are:*

1. *Depressive Reaction.* Derived from patient's responses at Year 8 to the question, "After an illness, even years after, some people may feel discouraged or depressed. Do you ever feel discouraged or depressed over your illness?"

2. *Gains from the Illness.* Based on patients' assessments in response to the question, "Despite all the problems and worries which your illness has involved over the years, do you see any possible gains or advantages coming out of this experience?"

3. *Change in Attitude toward Life.* The item draws on responses to the question, "Do you think your illness experience has made a difference in the way you think about life?"

4. *Achievement of Goals in Life.* This measure relies on self-assessment in response to the question, "How close do you think you have come to achieving life goals and ambitions you had when you were 21 years old?"

5. *Index of Symptoms.* This index is based on patients' self-report in regard to a series of 17 physiological and psychological symptom items.[1] Patients received a single-point score for each symptom experienced one or more times during the month preceding the Year 8 interview. The resulting distribution of total scores was

divided at the median into two categories: "high" and "low."

6. *Subjective Stress Scale.* As noted in Chapter 7, this index is based on patients' responses to four items which assess feelings of being under stress in usual life activities (Reeder et al., 1973). The resulting distribution was divided into terciles.[2] These are designated as "low," "medium," and "high," in regard to subjective stress at Year 8.

Analysis of Outcome at Year 8: The Total Population and Patients Classified by Severity of Illness. We carried out the analysis of outcome through two types of focus on the study population. We centered first upon (1) the patient group as a whole and second upon (2) the study group divided by a criterion of illness level: rehospitalization within 2 years prior to the Year 8 interview.

Some brief notes may be useful in regard to category (2). For purposes of analysis, our working assumption is that persons rehospitalized within a recent time period, such as 2 years, are more acutely ill and in less favorable condition from the actuarial standpoint than those who have not been rehospitalized during the period.

Accordingly, we classified patients on the basis of (1) reported rehospitalization for any cause during the 2 years prior to the Year 8 interview and (2) no rehospitalization within the 2 years. This second group includes men with a variety of health histories: those rehospitalized one or more times since Week 7 but not within the 2-year period prior to the Year 8 interview. It also includes those never rehospitalized.[3]

For the sake of brevity, in discussion of patients classified by health level we designated men in the first group as "Recently Hospitalized" (or "R-H"). The classification of "Not Recently Hospitalized" (or "Not R-H") applies to all other men.

The first approach, examination of the total patient population, permits answering core questions about the relationship of independent variables to dependent variables for the group as a whole. The second approach, dividing patients by severity of recent illness, designates populations whose needs *a priori* will differ. By separating the two groups by illness level, we can answer additional questions about ways in which these subgroups differ in terms of the social and psychological impact of the illness.

ANTECEDENTS AND CORRELATES OF OUTCOME AT YEAR 8

In examining the factors related to both the primary and secondary status indicators, two types of questions are pertinent: (1) What antecedent variables predict the primary and secondary status items at Year 8? and (2) What variables currently in the social, psychological, and situational spheres of patients are associated with the status index variables?

In centering on an 8-year time span, these questions concerning statistical relationships are linked to a number of larger issues to which the study as a whole is addressed. Thus, we attempt here to identify particular health, social, and psychological characteristics apparent in the early stages of a chronic illness which may have significant meaning for understanding a patient's subsequent long-term experience with the illness. A related series of questions is concerned with continuities in social integration and coping capacity. By enabling us to examine correlates at differing time points over a span of years our data permit some empirical documentation on these matters.

Another principal set of questions involves the problem of *current* correlates of the status or outcome variables 8 years after the first heart attack. Thus one of our main interests here is in the ways in which patterning of correlates occurs. We attempt to document the nature of association between these outcome variables in the later stages of a chronic illness. At the same time this approach may help develop "predictors" of patterns of outcome variables. Such knowledge can have some potential practical significance of course. For example, it may aid health planners in parsimonious attempts to designate target populations which may require special care, assistance, and supportive services.

Antecedents of Year 8 Status: Elements in the "Armory of Resources"

The Nature of the Variables.   For purposes of this research, data on antecedent variables are drawn from materials collected in the base-line study. They consist, in part, of items which describe the patient during the period before the first heart attack, at Week 7, and at Year 1.

In examining antecedent variables in relation to Year 8 outcome or status variables, we proceed in two ways in order to allow for flexibility in interpretation of the data. In the first, we consider the results in a primarily descriptive, relatively atheoretical fashion. In addition, we attempt to draw the data together through reference to the notion of "armory of resources," and to the functioning of particular types of resources and supports.

In line with these interests, we have included two types of variables in our analysis: those which in the usual sense cannot be considered as indicators of resources, such as demographic characteristics, and those which can represent actual resources and supports. Since the main thrust of our interpretation concerns resources, it may be useful here to specify further how they were operationalized for purposes of this research.

Throughout this volume, we have used the concept of the "armory of resources" as a frame of reference and as a means of organizing our description of the patients' long-term illness careers. Now in this chapter one of our main tasks is to examine various ways in which functioning of elements in the "armory of resources" may be related to long-term outcome. We start with the assumption that the elements classified as resources are part of the usual structure of supports potentially available to the men in the study population. This approach takes us beyond the question as to whether such elements as health, family, religious institutions, and agencies are resources. We assume that they are. Instead, we ask: In the case of the heart patient study population, what is the relative influence of various types of functioning of resources upon outcome? Which can best serve as "predictors?" Within which groups are they potentially most effective as "predictors?"

Measures of resources differ greatly in degree of specificity. For example, they range from appraisal of a condition such as level of marital happiness to a report on particular persons, "presence of a confidant." Such variability makes it difficult to describe in simple terms what the resource means in regard to outcome. The term "use" of a resource is misleading in that it implies possible conscious or active usage by the patient, and such a term is inappropriate in the sense that it cannot apply to "use of marital happiness" in the same sense that it does to "use of physician services."

Hence, in this chapter, when we look at possible relationships, we are guided by the concept of *function* as it is used in sociological analysis (Merton, 1957). Does presence of marital integration and high morale have consequences in terms of the outcomes for the heart patients in this study? In this exploratory study we cannot answer the question in as direct a manner as we would like. But we can determine whether antecedent measures of marital integration and morale are statistically related to our measures of social, psychological, and physical outcomes at Year 8. We can then make inferences about the meaning of such associations, insofar as the antecedents may have some functions or consequences for the phenomena which the outcome variables may measure.

We have operationalized our measures of resources or supports in the following ways. As we outlined in Chapter 1, the armory of resources is considered in this study in terms of three principal levels: (1) the individual, including physical health and emotional status; (2) larger institutional or social participation structures, such as family, church, work situation, informal social networks; and (3) formal organizations in the community, including institutions, agencies, the medical care organization, etc. The levels contain elements which overlap, of course, but they serve as means of differentiating three principal dimensions: those involving the individual and his internal resources, those of his personal social group and interaction system, and those at the level of the larger community and its organizations.

Within each of these levels we have selected a series of variables to serve as operational measures of resources or supports. The selection of these is based on evidence and/or theory in the social science literature regarding their actual or potential relevance to coping and adaptation. Thus, the variables may be classified as shown in Figure 8–1.

FIGURE 8–1.   OPERATIONAL MEASURES OF RESOURCES

I. Individual
    A. Health status variables

1. Physician ratings of functional health status at 1 year
2. Rehospitalization experience during first year
3. Patient reports of symptoms at earlier stages
B. Emotional status, psychological variables
    1. Psychological factors: emotional lability, ambition, and dominance
    2. Presence or absence of "coronary personality" characteristics
    3. Presence of early depressive reaction, predisposition to depression
    4. Subjective stress in base-line study
    5. Early positive morale
        Life satisfaction
        Perceived gains from the illness
        Positive change in attitude toward life
        Feeling of achievement of life's goals
II. Social
    A. Socioeconomic status
        1. Occupational level
        2. Educational Status
        3. Total Family Income
    B. Work role
        1. Perceptions of work in etiology
        2. Index of work stress
        3. Index of job dissatisfaction
        4. Frequency of lifting at work
    C. Family and friendship networks
        1. Family response to illness
        2. Stress of illness in other family members
        3. Marital status
        4. Marital happiness
        5. Index of marital disagreement
        6. Presence of a confidant
        7. Receipt of aid from family and quasi-kin
        8. Index of social participation
        9. Membership in clubs
    D. Religious organization and spiritual resources
        1. Religious affiliation
        2. Church attendance
        3. Importance of religion

III. Community and formal organizational systems
  A. Physician services
      1. Volume of visits
      2. Types of physicians visited
      3. Patient-physician relationship and continuity of care
      4. Areas of physician advice
      5. Compliance with the medical regimen
  B. Outpatient clinics, emergency rooms
  C. Use of hospital inpatient services: rehospitalizations of patients
  D. Utilization of other medical and social service professionals and agencies
  E. Institutional and organizational sources of income maintenance
      1. Social Security
      2. Health or disability insurance
      3. Veteran's benefits
      4. Unemployment compensation
      5. Retirement pensions

Use of the Variables in Analysis: Antecedents of Year 8 Statuses.   In our analysis we use items in the list of resource areas in Figure 8-1 to provide a means for examining questions or hypotheses concerning Year 8 outcome or status variables. In lieu of repeating each of the issues by rote, we will furnish some brief examples of the line of procedure.

Health status: physical. Our question for exploration postulates that positive health status functions as a resource, that over a long period patients with the most favorable physical health status initially will have more positive outcomes on the whole in terms of later health. As measures of health status, we employ physicians' ratings of the patients, level of physical symptoms, history of rehospitalization, and other measures.

Health status: emotional. Our working assumption is that patients with earlier evidence of emotional stability, good ego strength, and positive emotional tone will have more positive outcomes at Year 8 in terms of social and psychological measures. Among the antecedent measures which we can employ bearing on this matter are presence or absence of depressive reaction, indicators of mood, and reports of personal satisfaction with life and level of morale.

Family as resource. Among the various social supports which may influence long-term outcome, we assume that positive relationships in the family and kin group early in the illness experience will have favorable social and psychological effects evident at Year 8. We employ as measures such variables as reported presence of a confidant, evidence of aid and assistance from family members, and a positive marital relationship.

Further questions concerning patterning underlie our exploration of statistical relationships between antecedent variables and outcome. In what ways does the patterning reflect on the notion that patients who are socially integrated, who have good emotional stability, and who have an apparent network of supports are in the most favorable position for long-term positive outcomes? In what ways does the patterning enable us to designate target groups or subgroups within the population who may be particularly likely to have difficulties in long-term adaptation to the illness? These are questions and concerns which bring us to another important level of scrutiny of the findings on individual items.

Correlates of Statuses at Year 8: Current Resources and Supports

Here, we examine those resource phenomena existing concurrently with the Year 8 outcome measures. The resource variables are essentially the same as those listed in Figure 8-1, except that they are drawn from the time period current with the Year 8 interview. This approach to current resources and supports permits us to explore the pattern of their relationships with how well the patients are doing in regard to such matters as health, work, and general outlook at Year 8.

OUTCOME AND STATUSES AT YEAR 8: FINDINGS

Statuses of the Patients at Year 8: An Overview

The Primary Status Index Variables.   Table 8-1 presents data on the current statuses of patients in regard to work, health, and

Table 8-1. Primary Status Index Variables at Year 8. By Total Study
Population and by Recent Hospitalization Status.

| | | Recent Hospitalization Status | |
Primary Status Index Variable	Total Study Population*	Recently Hospitalized (R-H)	Not Recently Hospitalized (Not R-H)
Work-Retirement Status A			
Normal Career: In Work Force or Retired §	75.6	54.5[†]	85.2
Illness-Affected Career: Unemployed or Retired	24.4	45.5	14.8
Total Percent	100.0	100.0	100.0
Total N	205	66	135
Current Work Status B [‡]			
Employed	91.6	77.5[†]	96.4
Unemployed	8.4	22.5	3.6
Total Percent	100.0	100.0	100.0
Total N	154	40	110
Physician's Rating of Functional Health Status			
No Significant Impairment	65.7	47.0[†]	75.6
Moderate Impairment	14.3	16.3	13.3
Severe Impairment	20.0	36.7	11.1
Total Percent	100.0	100.0	100.0
Total N	140	49	90
Reported Satisfaction with Life			
Very Satisfied	26.7	27.6[†]	27.1
Satisfied	58.9	46.2	64.6
Not Satisfied	14.4	26.2	8.3
Total Percent	100.0	100.0	100.0
Total N	202	65	133

*Numbers for total N are affected by (a) exclusion of non-codable responses from patients and (b) number of physician ratings available. (See Note 2, Chapter 2.) The sum of the two health status cohorts is less than the total N because rehospitalization status of several patients was not codable due to non-response.

[†]On chi-square tests comparing the recently hospitalized and not recently hospitalized populations: p<.01.

[‡]Includes only men eligible for employment. Men no longer in the work force, such as those retired or disabled, are excluded.

§The term "Normal Career" simply refers to the absence of illness as a major factor affecting the work career.

life satisfaction at Year 8.[4] The table shows that physicians rated one-third of the patients as impaired to some degree. As we saw in Chapter 3, illness had removed a considerable proportion of patients from the work force, and a total of 25% were retired or currently out of work for health-related reasons. Patients generally reported that they were fairly satisfied with their current way of life. However, only about one-fourth described themselves as "very satisfied," while 60% rated themselves as "satisfied."

As might be expected, patients in the more severely ill category ("Recently Hospitalized") appeared to have a less favorable situation than those who had escaped rehospitalization in the previous 2 years. High proportions (46%) of the "R-H" men had left the work force for illness-related reasons and their doctors were more likely to have rated them as impaired to some degree (52%). One-fourth reported they were not satisfied with their current life situation.

These data have positive aspects which also deserve note. Among those recently hospitalized, over one-half were neither unemployed nor retired because of their illness, and nearly half were rated by their physicians as without significant impairment. Over one-fourth expressed high satisfaction with life, a proportion identical to that in the "Not R-H" group.

Some of the primary status index measures are interrelated, of course, as we shall later see in Table 8-3. Indeed, the work status of patients is in part determined by what their physicians advise. Reported satisfaction with life is related to both indices of work status. But the measures, while interrelated, do not appear to be infallible predictors of each other. For example, the physician's rating of functional health status and the patient's satifaction with life are not significantly associated.

The Secondary Status Index Variables.   Table 8-2 reports the distribution of patients' responses on each of the secondary status variables at Year 8.

Almost two-thirds saw some advantages or benefits in their illness, and over one-third indicated that the illness led them to have a more positive attitude toward life. About one-fourth of the patients reported a depressive reaction to the illness. A consider-

Table 8-2.   Secondary Status Index Variables at Year 8. By Total Study
Population and by Recent Hospitalization Status

		Recent Hospitalization Status	
Secondary Status Index Variable	Total Study Population[*]	Recently Hospitalized (R-H)	Not Recently Hospitalized (Not R-H)
Index of Symptoms[/]			
Low	59.0	54.5	61.5
High	41.0	45.5	38.5
Total Percent	100.0	100.0	100.0
Total N	205	66	135
Subjective Stress Scale[/]			
Low	38.4	34.8	40.6
Medium	36.5	33.3	37.6
High	25.1	31.8	21.8
Total Percent	100.0	100.0	100.0
Total N	203	66	133
Depressive Reaction to the Illness			
Yes	24.4	36.4[a]	17.8
No	75.6	63.6	82.2
Total Percent	100.0	100.0	100.0
Total N	205	66	135
Perceived Gains From the Illness			
Yes	59.8	50.0[b]	64.2
No	40.2	50.0	35.8
Total Percent	100.0	100.0	100.0
Total N	204	66	134
Change in Attitude Toward Life			
Positive	37.6	30.3[c]	41.5
No Change	44.4	43.9	44.4
Other Than Positive	18.0	25.8	14.1
Total Percent	100.0	100.0	100.0
Total N	205	66	135

able proportion (43%) felt they had fallen behind in achieving their life goals.

Contrary to our expectations, we found few marked differences between those who were hospitalized and those who were not hospitalized in the preceding 2 years. The two groups differ

Table 8-2 (Continued)

| | | Recent Hospitalization Status | |
Secondary Status Index Variable	Total Study Population*	Recently Hospitalized (R-H)	Not Recently Hospitalized (Not R-H)
Achievement of Life Goals			
Achievement Beyond Early Goals	14.5	16.7	13.9
Achievement Matches Early Goals	42.5	38.3	45.1
Fallen Behind in Achievement of Goals	43.0	45.0	41.0
Total Percent	100.0	100.0	100.0
Total N	186	60	122

*Numbers for total N vary due to exclusion of non-codable reponses from patients. The sum of the two health status cohorts is less than the total N because rehospitalization status of several patients was not codable.

†The Index of Symptoms and Subjective Stress Scale are additive indices developed by combining responses to several individual items. See text and Note 2.

a = p<.01.

b = p<.05.

c = p<.10.

somewhat but not significantly in their distributions on the series of variables. A significantly higher percentage of those recently hospitalized reported depressive reaction at Year 8 and perceived no gains as a result of their illness. Recency of hospitalization was not associated with any of the other items—quality of life, symptoms, or subjective stress, although suggestive trends in the direction of significance appeared.

Of most interest, perhaps, is the finding that many of the recently hospitalized men reported the overall quality of their lives as favorable, while numerous patients free of recent acute illness reported more negative perceptions of their lives. Half of the "R-H" patients believed there were gains from their illness and 30% reported the illness had led to positive changes in their attitude toward life. Over a third of these men were in the "low subjective stress" group, a proportion nearly matching that of men who were "Not R-H." At the same time, the current lives of the "Not R-H" patients appeared to have many unhappy aspects, as reflected in part in reports of dissatisfaction with life and failure in achieving life goals. The proportion of these men who scored "high" on the index of symptoms is not significantly lower than that of the"R-H" group. Thus, for the heart patient population as a whole, apparent severity of the illness was not the critical factor in life satisfaction and quality of life at Year 8.

Primary and Secondary Status Variables: Interrelations.   Table 8–3 shows various interrelations between primary and secondary status index measures at Year 8. Reports of depressive reaction, for example, are related to low morale as represented by patients' negative change in their views of life and feelings of nonachievement of life goals. As might be expected, depressive reaction is associated with lack of satisfaction with the current life situation. Patients with depressive reaction are also likely to report high symptoms and high subjective stress.

Further examination of Table 8–3 reveals that the secondary status variables in general are associated most strongly with subjective reports of satisfaction with life. Particular secondary measures, however, also relate to two other primary status indices, work-retirement status A and physician assessments. An "illness-affected" work status, for example, was associated with frequent reports of symptoms and illness-related depressive reaction at Year 8. An "impaired" rating by the physician at Year 8 was related to high scores on the Index of Symptoms, reports of depressive reaction, and few perceived advantages of the illness.

Such interrelations do more than lend support for the face validity of our main measures. The matrix of interrelations helps provide a composite empirical portrayal of ways in which the problems of heart patients in one life area may relate to problems in other spheres.

Antecedents of Outcome at Year 8: Findings

We now turn to our major focus in this chapter, as we examine a series of antecedent variables and their sequelae at Year 8.

Table 8-3. Associations Among Status Index Variables at Year 8.
Gamma Scores and Levels of Significance as Indicated
by Chi-Square Test*

Status Index Variables	1a	1b	2	3	4	5	6	7	8
Primary Variables									
1a. Work-Retirement Status A: Normal/Illness-Affected									
1b. Current Work Status B: Employed/Unemployed	NA								
2. Physician's Rating of Functional Health Status	.63[a]	NS							
3. Reported Satisfaction with Life	.46[a]	.87[a]	NS						
Secondary Variables									
4. Index of Symptoms	-.47[a]	NS	-.50[a]	-.57[a]					
5. Subjective Stress Scale	NS	NS	NS	-.39[a]	.40[a]				
6. Depressive Reaction	-.52[a]	NS	-.48[a]	-.67[a]	.52[a]	.48[a]			
7. Perceived Gains from the Illness	NS	NS	.23[b]	.46[a]	-.35[b]	NS	-.58[a]		
8. Positive Changes in Attitude	NS	NS	NS	.42[a]	-.38[a]	NS	-.39[a]	.51[a]	
9. Achievement of Life Goals	NS	NS	NS	.61[a]	NS	-.39[a]	-.39[b]	NS	.27[a]

*N = 205. The N for each gamma score varies due to the omission of "no response," "not relevant," and "don't know" responses.

a,b: On chi-square test of significance, a = p<.01, b = p<.05.

NS = not significant on chi-square test or no meaningful relationship indicated by gamma scores.

NA = not applicable.

219

Tracing the surviving patient population over the years, several characteristics of the patients from the base-line study appear to be related to status variables at Year 8. These antecedent variables are mainly: (1) health measures; (2) indicators of emotional strain or work stress; and (3) some measures of the quality and perceived meaning of life. Further, some notable relationships involving pre-illness occupation emerged, particularly in regard to the semiskilled and unskilled. However, social status characteristics, age, and other antecedent measures drawn from work, family, and the like, generally did not exhibit comparable patterns of significant statistical relationships with statuses at Year 8.

As Table 8–4 shows, physician ratings of patients' functional health status at Year 1 were related to several areas examined at Year 8: (1) work-retirement status; (2) level of symptoms; and (3) reported depressive reaction. The relationship between early physician ratings and depressive reaction at Year 8 was more marked for the "R-H" than for the "Not R-H" group. In addition, although statistical significance is not present, some long-term suggestive trends can be seen in the table. In particular, these appear in data relating the Year 1 physician assessment to measures of morale 7 years later, such as life satisfaction, a positive change in outlook on life, and perceived gains from the illness.

In our earlier book, *The Heart Patient Recovers* (Croog & Levine, 1977), we had noted the long-term association between early indicators of health problems (Week 7) and subsequent ratings of health 1 year later. In a consistent fashion, the physician rating at Year 1 is also related to later problems at Year 8, such as illness-associated interruption of the work career, depressive reaction, and poor morale. At first impression, we might conclude that the pattern here may be one in which health measures appear to be related over time primarily because they describe the same underlying and continuing phenomenon of illness. Early poor health is reflected in health-related problems years later. However, the phenomena are more complex than such an interpretation would indicate, and obviously, additional illnesses and recoveries over the study period must also be taken into account.

It also appears from Table 8–4 that, for the total population, early indicators of emotional strain, such as depressive reaction and subjective stress, are related at Year 8 to level of reported symptoms, subjective stress, and depressive reaction, as well as to perceptions of the meaning of life and achievement of life goals. Moreover, when we compare the "R-H" and the "Not R-H" groups the results are essentially the same as for the total population, suggesting similar underlying patterns in both groups. The one exception is "subjective stress." A series of meaningful associations appear only among the "Not R-H" linking subjective stress at Week 7 and Year 1 with subjective stress at Year 8.

These findings are on the whole consistent with the data reported in Chapter 7, particularly with reference to the series of self-rated psychological characteristics. Several ratings of pre-illness psychological items at Week 7 were related to analogous Year 8 measures. Items assessing emotional lability exhibited continuity over time, and as we will see, these pre-illness characteristics were related to the Subjective Stress Scale at Year 8 as well (Table 8-5).

Finally, as Table 8-4 shows, items in the base-line study which measured perceived quality of life were related to similar measures later at Year 8. Feelings of achievement of life goals and optimistic belief in the constructive aspects of illness at Week 7 and Year 1 were associated with subsequent life satisfaction, feelings of achievement of goals, favorable views of the meaning of the illness, and absence of depressive reaction. This is a major emergent theme for the total population, and similar patterns appear when "R-H" and "Not R-H" groups are compared.

Some initially perplexing elements in these data also deserve note. Physician rating at Year 1 is not statistically related to physician rating at Year 8 for the total population of survivors. However, other measures of the health of survivors at Year 8, as we noted, are related to the corresponding Year 1 rating. In other words, "patient-derived" data at Year 1 and Year 8 are related, but "physician-derived" data are not. The explanation lies not in the adequacy of physician judgment, but in the nature of the distribution in cells. For example, only 13 men rated as limited in activities at Year 1 were rated the same way at Year 8. A three-category distribution of this group for analysis produced inadequate numbers in cells for meaningful results on the chi-square test.[5]

The utility of the physician measure of functional health

Table 8-4. Associations Between Antecedent Variables and Year 8 Status Index Variables. By Total Study Population and by Recent Hospitalization Status. Gamma Scores and Levels of Significance as Indicated by Chi-Square Test.*

	Primary Status Variables			Secondary Status Variables					
Antecedent Variables	Work-Retirement Status At	Physician's Rating of Functional Health Status	Reported Satisfaction With Life	Index of Symptoms	Subjective Stress Scale	Depressive Reaction	Perceived Gains From the Illness	Positive Change in Attitude	Achievement of Life Goals
SOCIAL IDENTITY VARIABLES:									
Age at Week 7									
Total	$-.38^b$	--	--	$.25^c$	--	--	--	--	--
Recently Hospitalized	--	x	x	x	x	x	x	x	x
Not Recently Hospitalized#	$-.48^c$	x	--	$.30^c$	--	--	--	--	--
Educational Level									
Total	$.19^d$	--	--	$-.20^d$	--	--	$.22^c$	--	--
R-H	--	x	x	--	--	--	--	--	x
Not R-H	--	x	x	--	--	--	$.26^d$	--	--
Pre-Illness Occupation (Blue Collar, White Collar)									
Total	--	--	--	$-.23^d$	--	--	$.52^a$	$.36^a$	--
R-H	--	x	x	--	$-.43^c$	$-.62^b$	$.61^b$	x	x
Not R-H	--	x	--	--	$.40^b$	--	$.47^b$	$.29^a$	--

222

Table 8-4 (Continued)

Antecedent Variables	Primary Status Variables			Secondary Status Variables					
	Work-Retirement Status A/	Physician's Rating of Functional Health Status	Reported Satisfaction With Life	Index of Symptoms	Subjective Stress Scale	Depressive Reaction	Perceived Gains From the Illness	Positive Change in Attitude	Achievement of Life Goals
Pre-Illness Occupation (4 Levels)									
Total	--	x	--	$-.27^c$	--	--	$.30^a$	$.27^a$	--
R-H	x	x	--	x	x	x	x	x	x
Not R-H	x	x	x	$-.30^d$	--	--	$.29^c$	x	x
Year 8 Occupation (4 Levels)									
Total	$.38^d$	x	x	--	x	--	$.40^a$	x	x
R-H	x	x	x	x	x	x	x	x	x
Not R-H	x	x	x	--	x	x	$.45^b$	x	x
WEEK 7 ANTECEDENT VARIABLES:									
Achievement of Life Goals									
Total	--	--	$.37^b$	--	--	--	--	--	$.61^a$
R-H	--	x	x	$-.39^b$	x	--	$.39^d$	--	x
Not R-H	--	x	x	--	$-.23^d$	--	--	--	$.55^a$
Perceived Gains From the Illness									
Total	$.31^c$	$.21^d$	$.38^a$	$-.47^a$	--	$-.38^b$	$.67^a$	$.35^a$	--
R-H	--	x	$.50^b$	$-.51^b$	--	$-.42^d$	$.56^b$	$.48^b$	$.37^c$
Not R-H	--	x	--	$-.39^b$	--	--	$.70^a$	--	--

223

8-4 (Continued)

	Primary Status Variables			Secondary Status Variables					
Antecedent Variables	Work-Retirement Status At	Physician's Rating of Functional Health Status	Reported Satisfaction With Life	Index of Symptoms	Subjective Stress Scale	Depressive Reaction	Perceived Gains From the Illness	Positive Change in Attitude	Achievement of Life Goals
Week 7 Subjective Stress Items									
Nervous Strain in Daily Activities									
Total	--	--	$-.23^d$	--	$.40^a$	--	--	--	--
R-H	--	x	--	--	$.30^d$	--	--	--	--
Not R-H	--	x	$-.36^b$	--	$.44^a$	--	--	--	--
Generally Tense and Nervous									
Total	--	$-.25^d$	--	$.21^d$	$.30^b$	$.25^d$	--	--	--
R-H	--	x	--	--	--	--	$.39^d$	$.21^d$	$.26^d$
Not R-H	--	--	--	$.27^d$	$.38^b$	--	--	--	--
YEAR 1 ANTECEDENT VARIABLES:									
Physician's Rating of Functional Health Status									
Total	$.39^a$	--	$.28^c$	$-.43^a$	--	$-.37^b$	$.27^d$	$.32^c$	--
R-H	$.48^c$	x	x	x	x	$-.50^b$	x	x	x
Not R-H	--	x	--	x	x	--	--	x	x
Marital Happiness									
Total	--	x	$.32^b$	--	--	--	--	--	--
R-H	--	x	x	--	x	--	--	x	x
Not R-H	--	x	x	--	--	--	$.20^b$	--	--

Table 8-4 (Continued)

Antecedent Variables	Primary Status Variables			Secondary Status Variables					
	Work-Retirement Status A7	Physician's Rating of Functional Health Status	Reported Satisfaction with Life	Index of Symptoms	Subjective Stress Scale	Depressive Reaction	Perceived Gains From the Illness	Positive Change in Attitude	Achievement of Life Goals
Index of Social Participation									
Total	--	$.28^{d}$	--	--	--	$-.35^{b}$	--	--	--
R-H	--	$.52^{c}$	--	--	--	--	--	--	--
Not R-H	--	x	--	--	--	$-.60^{a}$	--	$-.21^{c}$	--
Frequency of Walks									
Total	$-.34^{d}$	--	--	$-.24^{d}$	--	--	--	--	--
R-H	--	x	--	--	--	--	--	$-.34^{d}$	x
Not R-H	--	x	$.26^{d}$	$-.38^{b}$	--	--	$.30^{d}$	$.24^{d}$	--
Achievement of Life Goals									
Total	--	--	$.37^{a}$	--	$-.21^{d}$	--	--	--	$.54^{a}$
R-H	--	x	$.46^{b}$	--	$-.46^{b}$	--	--	--	x
Not R-H	--	x	x	--	--	--	--	--	$.48^{a}$
Perceived Gains From the Illness									
Total	--	$.30^{d}$	$.22^{d}$	$-.24^{d}$	--	$-.25^{d}$	$.71^{a}$	--	--
R-H	--	x	--	--	--	--	$.67^{a}$	--	--
Not R-H	--	--	--	$-.33^{c}$	--	--	$.74^{a}$	--	--

225

Table 8-4 (Continued)

Antecedent Variables	Primary Status Variables			Secondary Status Variables					
	Work-Retirement Status A	Physician's Rating of Functional Health Status	Reported Satisfaction With Life	Index of Symptoms	Subjective Stress Scale	Depressive Reaction	Perceived Gains From the Illness	Positive Change in Attitude	Achievement of Life Goals
Depressive Reaction									
Total	--	$-.32^d$	--	$.34^b$	$.30^b$	$.51^a$	--	--	$-.35^b$
R-H	--	x	$-.31^d$	$.43^a$	--	$.65^a$	--	--	$-.56^b$
Not R-H	$-.46^c$	--	--	$.31^d$	$.35^b$	$.49^b$	--	--	$-.26^d$
Index of Work Stress									
Total	--	--	$-.20^c$	$.27^d$	$.34^a$	$.40^a$	$-.28^c$	--	--
R-H	--	x	$-.36^d$	--	--	$.48^c$	$-.41^d$	--	x
Not R-H	--	x	--	$.30^d$	$.37^a$	--	$-.20^d$	--	--
Year 1 Subjective Stress Items									
Nervous Strain in Daily Activities									
Total	--	--	--	$.31^b$	$.27^b$	$.32^c$	--	--	--
R-H	--	--	--	$.40^d$	--	--	--	$-.29^d$	--
Not R-H	--	--	--	$.26^d$	$.37^b$	--	--	--	--
Generally Tense and Nervous									
Total	--	--	$-.31^b$	$.26^c$	$.28^c$	$.42^a$	--	--	--
R-H	--	--	--	--	--	--	--	--	--
Not R-H	$-.49^c$	--	$-.28^c$	--	$.43^a$	$.52^b$	--	--	--

226

Table 8-4 (Continued)

*For listing of coding values of variables, see Appendix D.

Total N = 205. Recently Hospitalized N = 66, Not Recently Hospitalized N = 137. Numbers for total N are affected by (a) number of physician ratings available and (b) exclusion of noncodable responses from patients (see Note 2, Chapter 2). Because two respondents' recent hospitalization status was unclassified due to nonresponse, the sum of the two health-status cohorts is less than the total N.

a = p<.01, b = p<.05, c = p<.10, d = p<.20.
-- = Not significant on chi-square test or no meaningful relationship indicated by gamma score.
x = Expected value less than 5 in more than 20% of cells; chi-square and gamma not computed.

†Reports on crosstabulations involving Current Work Status B (employed vs. unemployed) are omitted from this table, since only a small number of nonretired men were unemployed at Year 8. Numbers were too few for systematic review of relationships between antecedent variables and this outcome variable.

#Hereafter, for the sake of brevity, the illness level categories will be designated as R-H and Not R-H.

227

status at Year 1 as a possible predictor does appear to be borne out, as we explained in Chapter 2, when long-term health outcomes are examined. Here the numbers were clearly sufficient for analysis. As we saw, a significant association emerged between the physician's assessment of the patient at Year 1 and later occurrence of death and/or rehospitalization due to heart disease.

When we apply the "armory of resources" framework as a point of reference for summarizing data in the table, a congruent pattern emerges. First, there appear to be distinctive statistical continuities in health level, emotional status, morale, and outlook on life. The patient who is ill at Year 1 as characterized by his physician, is particularly likely to be troubled subsequently by physical and emotional problems. Patients who describe themselves as emotionally labile, stressed, and anxious at Year 1 tend to display the same patterns at Year 8. Those who exhibit personal resilience and a positive outlook on life at Year 1 manifest the same qualities at Year 8. Thus, the antecedent resource variables which seem most influential in their associations with later positive outcome are a favorable health rating by the physician, absence of emotional strain, and maintenance of good morale. Higher occupational status also seemed to function as a resource variable, judging by its association with some indicators of positive morale at Year 8, such as perception of gains from the illness.

Using our system of "controls," patients were categorized by severity of illness, "R-H" and "Not R-H." Within each group patterns similar to those found for the total population tended to prevail. Early indicators of emotional strain, morale, and quality of life appeared to be useful predictors of these same states of mind 7 years later in both groups of men. Nevertheless, some differences between the two groups did emerge.

For example, the relationship between physician ratings at Year 1 and depressive reaction at Year 8 was especially marked for the "R-H" men. Thus, for this group in particular, depressive feelings might have been predicted on the basis of earlier information about the severity of their illness. Such differences between the two groups might be explained by the fact that the "R-H" group had more health problems at Year 8 than the "Not R-H" men, and thus had more basis for depressive reaction and lower morale.

We also note in Table 8-4 a general lack of association between Year 8 status variables and earlier social and demographic measures from the pre-illness and Year 8 periods. Aside from those already discussed, other antecedent variables relating to social structural, situational, and interpersonal interaction did not generally appear to be associated with outcomes. This does not mean, of course, that no associations exist; we can only conclude that our data do not reveal them.

In contrast, the several items in Table 8-4 which pertain in particular to physical health, emotional state, and morale exhibit an apparently inexorable quality. Regardless of factors external to the individual, these core characteristics seem to manifest a continuity of their own. This pattern is consistent with principles of personality theory regarding the persistence of basic ego structure and defense mechanisms. As many have pointed out, how the person deals with situations is strongly influenced by ego structure or "basic personality." The case can be made that by implication, the data in Table 8-4 are consistent with this theme.

If the principal findings in the table are the product of continuities, it may be possible early to designate target groups which are particularly likely to require care, in terms of both their physical and emotional health. For example, if the findings reported here could have been systematically applied at Year 1 in a prospective manner, many of the stresses awaiting patients and their families might have been alleviated through appropriate supports and services of professionals and agencies. Some of the ramifications of this prospect for practitioners, health-care planners, patients, and their families are reviewed in Chapter 9.

Ratings of Pre-Illness Psychological Characteristics and Outcome at Year 8

The possible relationship between patients' psychological characteristics and long-term health outcomes was examined by means of their self-perceptions. As we explained in Chapter 7, at Week 7 men assessed their pre-illness psychological characteristics on a list of 22 items. These data were subjected to a principal component type factor analysis in order to determine simple structure. Three factors were extracted, and factor scores on each were computed for each patient. These three sets of factor

Table 8-5. Associations Between Pre-Illness Psychological Factors (Rated at Week 7) and Year 8 Status Index Variables: Total Study Population and by Recent Hospitalization Status. Gamma Scores and Levels of Significance as Indicated by Chi-Square Test*

Pre-Illness Psychological Factor	Primary Status Variables			Secondary Status Variables					
	Work-Retirement Status A†	Physician's Rating of Functional Health Status	Reported Satisfaction With Life	Index of Symptoms	Subjective Stress Scale	Depressive Reaction	Perceived Gains From the Illness	Positive Change in Attitude	Achievement of Life Goals
Emotional Lability									
Total	-.28^c	--	-.28^b	.26^b	.44^a	.36^a	--	--	-.21^d
R-H‡	-.24^b	x	--	.29^a	.38^d	--	--	--	x
Not R-H	-.34^b	x	-.33^b	--	.48^a	.39^a	--	--	-.28^d
Ambition									
Total	--	--	--	--	--	--	--	--	--
R-H	--	x	.28^d	--	.33^d	-.30^d	--	--	x
Not R-H	--	x	x	--	--	--	--	--	.23^d
Dominance									
Total	--	--	--	--	--	--	--	.25^b	--
R-H	-.36^d	x	--	--	--	-.40^d	--	--	x
Not R-H	--	x	x	--	.32^c	--	--	.28^d	--

230

Table 8-5 (Continued)

*For listing of coding values of variables, see Appendix D. Factor scores were grouped in terciles for purposes of analysis.

Total N = 205. Recently Hospitalized N =66, Not Recently Hospitalized N = 137. Numbers for total N are affected by (a) number of physician ratings available and (b) exclusion of noncodable responses from patients (see Note 2, Chapter 2). Because two respondents' recent hospitalization status was unclassified due to nonresponse, the sum of the two health status cohorts is less than the total N.

a = $p<.01$, b = $p<.05$, c = $p<.10$, d = $p<.20$
-- = Not significant on chi-square test or no meaningful relationship indicated by gamma score.
x = Expected value less than 5 in more than 20 percent of cells; chi-square and gamma not computed.

[†]Numbers were too few for systematic review of relationships between pre-illness psychological factors and Current Work Status B. See Note [†] in Table 8-4.

[‡] R-H = Recently Hospitalized, Not R-H = Not Recently Hospitalized.

231

scores were then divided into terciles, roughly designated as high, medium, and low.

For the total population, as seen in Table 8-5, scores on pre-illness "emotional lability" were positively associated with an illness-affected work career, and high subjective stress, symptoms, and depressive reaction at Year 8. They were negatively associated with satisfaction with life. When controls for illness level were introduced, a similar pattern of results emerged for both "R-H" and "Not R-H" men with regard to work career and subjective stress.

However, the two groups differed in other areas. For the "R-H" men, pre-illness "emotional lability" was not related to measures of morale and emotional state at Year 8. For the "Not R-H," however, suggestive relationships appear linking pre-illness "emotional lability" with morale and emotional state 8 years later. Men who were free from recent hospitalization exhibited a pattern of relationship between high scores on "emotional lability" and Year 8 reports of depressive reaction, dissatisfaction with life, subjective stress, and failure to achieve goals in life. These data imply that those with the least severe illness course, the pre-illness psychological factor of "emotional lability" may help "predict" later morale and emotional state.[6]

The other psychological factors "ambition" and "dominance" were not significantly associated with Year 8 status variables, although several suggestive findings appear in the table.

Viewed in the context of the "armory of resources" these findings on self-perceptions of pre-illness psychological characteristics may have implications for understanding patients' subsequent health histories. In particular, the psychological characteristics associated with "emotional lability" seemed to be related to several key areas of subsequent experience, and those patients with early "high" emotional lability seemed most likely at Year 8 to have problems of general morale, i.e., low life satisfaction, reported depressive reaction, frequent symptoms, and high subjective stress. It was thus "better" to be initially equipped with high emotional stability, not subject to depression, nervousness, excitement, or sensitivity to personal affront.

These findings are even more marked for the least seriously ill—the "Not Recently Hospitalized." What does this mean? Why are relationships between early emotional status and later morale less marked among the more seriously ill (R-H) than for the least seriously ill (Not R-H)? For those most seriously ill, as we suggested in *The Heart Patient Recovers* (Croog & Levine, 1977), the sheer fact of physical illness may override earlier factors of a psychological or social nature. However, among those who have not experienced a recent illness crisis, early psychological factors may be more important in influencing morale, mode of coping, and view of life. That these phenomena may be observable over an 8-year period is most noteworthy.

Current Correlates of Outcome at Year 8: Findings

The discussion thus far has centered on status or outcome measures at Year 8, principally in relation to various *antecedent* variables. We turn now to another issue, the possible association of *current* social and psychological characteristics with Year 8 status variables. In other words, at the time of Year 8 what was the pattern of association between patients' characteristics and their concurrent outcome traits?

When variables drawn from the Year 8 interview were examined in relation to Year 8 status measures, several consistent patterns of association emerged (see Table 8-6). Most were in line with what might be expected, given the findings we have already reported. For example, reported marital happiness was related to satisfaction with life, aspects of positive morale, and low subjective stress. Similarly, marital disagreement was negatively related to life satisfaction and positively associated with reported subjective stress and depressive reaction.

Patients who had a confidant at Year 8 also were most likely to report satisfaction with life, few symptoms, low subjective stress, and absence of depressive reaction. Measures of religious behavior and belief, such as church attendance and high valuation of religion, were found to be related to perceptions of gains resulting from the illness. Further, reported work stress and job dissatisfaction appeared to be negatively associated with satisfaction with life and perceived achievement of life goals, and they were positively related to reported total symptoms, subjective

Table 8-6. Associations Between Year 8 Variables and Year 8 Status Index Variables. By Total Population and by Recent Hospitalization Status. Gamma Scores and Levels of Significance as Indicated by Chi-Square Test*

Year 8 Variables	Primary Status Variables			Secondary Status Variables					
	Work-Retirement Status At	Physician's Rating of Functional Health Status	Reported Satisfaction With Life	Index of Symptoms	Subjective Stress Scale	Depressive Reaction	Perceived Gains From the Illness	Positive Change in Attitude	Achievement of Life Goals
Total Family Income									
Total	.55^d	x	x	-.39^a	--	-.23^d	.20^d	-.24^c	x
R-H†	x	x	x	--	x	x	x	x	x
Not R-H	x	x	x	-.45^a	--	x	--	x	x
Marital Status									
Total	--	x	.37^c	--	--	--	--	--	--
R-H	--	x	x	--	x	--	--	x	--
Not R-H	--	x	x	-.39^d	--	--	--	.40^a	--
Marital Happiness									
Total	--	--	.57^a	--	-.27^b	--	.37^a	.28^c	.32^c
R-H	--	x	.46^c	--	--	--	--	x	x
Not R-H	--	x	x	--	--	--	.48^a	.35^c	--
Index of Marital Disagreement									
Total	--	--	-.33^b	--	.34^a	.38^a	--	--	--
R-H	--	x	-.34^d	--	.33^a	--	--	x	x
Not R-H	.29^c	x	x	--	.36^a	.56^a	--	x	--

Table 8-6 (Continued)

	Primary Status Variables			Secondary Status Variables					
Year 8 Variables	Work-Retirement Status At	Physician's Rating of Functional Health Status	Reported Satisfaction With Life	Index of Symptoms	Subjective Stress Scale	Depressive Reaction	Perceived Gains From the Illness	Positive Change in Attitude	Achievement of Life Goals
Index of Social Participation									
Total	--	--	--	--	--	-.37[b]	.23[d]	--	--
R-H	--	x	--	-.38[d]	--	-.67[a]	--	--	--
Not R-H	--	-.31[a]	--	--	--	--	.34[c]	--	--
Membership in Clubs									
Total	.27[d]	.27[b]	.29[b]	--	--	--	.27[c]	.25[d]	.27[a]
R-H	--	x	x	--	x	x	x	x	x
Not R-H	--	--	x	--	--	--	.29[a]	--	--
Presence of Confidant									
Total	--	--	.52[a]	-.35[c]	-.50[a]	-.45[b]	--	--	--
R-H	--	x	x	--	-.74[a]	-.59[c]	--	--	x
Not R-H	--	x	.42[b]	-.51[b]	-.39[c]	-.42[d]	--	--	--
Church Attendance									
Total	--	--	.29[c]	-.27[b]	--	--	.32[b]	--	--
R-H	--	x	--	--	--	--	.44[b]	--	x
Not R-H	--	x	x	-.37[b]	--	--	--	--	--

235

Table 8-6 (Continued)

	Primary Status Variables			Secondary Status Variables					
Year 8 Variables	Work-Retirement Status A†	Physician's Rating of Functional Health Status	Reported Satisfaction With Life	Index of Symptoms	Subjective Stress Scale	Depressive Reaction	Perceived Gains From the Illness	Positive Change in Attitude	Achievement of Life Goals
Importance of Religion									
Total	--	--	.37[b]	--	--	--	.35[b]	--	--
R-H	--	x	.38[d]	--	--	--	.56[b]	--	--
Not R-H	--	x	--	--	--	--	--	--	--
Frequency of Walks									
Total	--	--	.26[c]	--	-.23[b]	-.27[c]	.34[a]	--	--
R-H	--	x	x	x	x	--	x	x	x
Not R-H	--	x	--	--	--	-.35[b]	.37[b]	--	--
Frequency of Lifting on the Job									
Total	--	x	--	--	--	x	-.37[c]	-.21[d]	--
R-H	x	x	x	x	x	x	x	x	x
Not R-H	x	x	--	.41[c]	--	--	-.47[b]	-.26[c]	x
Index of Work Stress									
Total	x	x	-.30[b]	.31[c]	.65[a]	.31[a]	--	--	--
R-H	x	x	x	x	x	x	x	x	x
Not R-H	x	x	x	--	.66[a]	.48[a]	--	.31[a]	--

236

Table 8-6 (Continued)

Year 8 Variables	Primary Status Variables			Secondary Status Variables					
	Work-Retirement Status A‡	Physician's Rating of Functional Health Status	Reported Satisfaction With Life	Index of Symptoms	Subjective Stress Scale	Depressive Reaction	Perceived Gains From the Illness	Positive Change in Attitude	Achievement of Life Goals
Index of Job Dis-satisfaction									
Total	x	--	-.71a	.27d	.49a	.53a	--	--	-.42b
R-H	x	x	x	x	x	x	x	x	x
Not R-H	x	x	x	--	.49a	.53a	--	--	-.36d

*For listing of coding values of variables, see Appendix D.

Total N = 205. Recently Hospitalized N = 66, Not Recently Hospitalized N = 137. Numbers for total N are affected by (a) number of physician ratings available and (b) exclusion of noncodable responses from patients (see Note 2, Chapter 2). Because two respondents' recent hospitalization status was unclassified due to nonresponse, the sum of the two health status cohorts is less than the total N.

$a = p<.01$, $b = p<.05$, $c = p<.10$, $d = p<.20$.

-- Not significant on chi-square test or no meaningful relationship indicated by gamma score.

x = Expected value less than 5 in more than 20 percent of cells; chi-square and gamma not computed.

†Numbers were too few for systematic review of relationships between Year 8 variables and Current Work Status B. See Note† in Table 8-4.

‡R-H = Recently Hospitalized, Not R-H = Not Recently Hospitalized.

stress, and depressive reaction. Other data exhibited the same general pattern.

On the whole, demographic and social status variables did not emerge as strong correlates of status at Year 8.

Comparison of the "R-H" and "Not R-H" groups with regard to correlates of Year 8 status is handicapped by small numbers in cells. Nevertheless, some suggestive themes appear. In general, the data for both groups of patients reveal a pattern which is consistent with that of the total population. There were some interesting exceptions, however.

In some instances, relationships between Year 8 correlates and statuses apparent in the total population were strengthened when controls for severity of illness were introduced. For example, relationships between variables assessing the quality of the marital relationship and aspects of patient morale were especially consistent for the "Not R-H" men. Associations between reported work stress and job dissatisfaction and (1) subjective stress, and (2) depressive reaction were apparent only for the "Not R-H." On the other hand, the presence of a confidant seemed to be more highly associated with low subjective stress and absence of depressive reaction among the "R-H" than the "Not R-H" men. The finding which linked religious attitudes and behavior and perceptions of gains from the illness appeared only for the "R-H" patients. Thus, among the most ill men in particular, availability of a confidant and religious supports appeared to make a difference in outlook and emotional state.

Considering these materials with reference to the "armory of resources," high consistency is apparent between the patterns just described, and earlier data on antecedent variables and outcome at Year 8. For example, low work stress and satisfaction with one's job at Year 8 were associated with several concurrent outcome measures, including few reported symptoms and positive morale. Of particular interest is the consistent association between current social supports and measures of social integration in relation to outcome at Year 8. For example, the presence of a confidant, indicators of marital integration, and to a lesser extent, some measures of social participation appear to form a pattern of positive relationship to outcome.

Summary

This chapter has examined relationships between (1) outcome at 8 years after a first myocardial infarction, and (2) previous and current social, psychological, and demographic characteristics of the patients. We first reviewed two sets of variables serving as operational indices of outcome. Measures of "statuses" in major life areas at Year 8 comprised the indices. The *primary status index variables* consisted of measures of participation in the work force, physicians' ratings of health status, and patients' satisfaction with life. The *secondary status index variables* supplemented the primary measures, drawing upon reports by patients concerning various other aspects of their lives.

As we expected, higher proportions of those most recently ill had either left the work force or had been rated lowest in functional capacity by their physicians. Significantly, more rated themselves as not satisfied with their current lives than did those men who had not suffered an acute illness episode within the last 2 years. Data for the secondary status index variables showed as well that recent severity of illness was related to current depressive reaction in this population of men, and there were some suggestive associations between illness status and morale measures. Equally impressive, however, were the percentages within the groups indicating positive reactions among many of the most ill and negative reactions among the least ill.

In regard to associations between antecedent characteristics of patients and outcomes at Year 8, several principal themes emerged. (1) Between Year 1 and Year 8, there were continuities in patients' reports of their emotional status and their views concerning the meaning and quality of life. Early depressive reaction, subjective stress, and measures of morale and personal outlook on life were associated with responses on similar items 7 years later. (2) Early physicians' ratings of patients' health were related to later work status, symptom levels, and depressive reactions, and there were suggestive trends in relationship of the ratings to patients' satisfaction with life and view of life at Year 8. (3) Measures of subjective stress and work stress at Year 1 were associated with patient reports of symptoms and depressive reaction at Year 8. (4) Occupational level before the first heart attack appeared to be related to some measures of morale 8 years later. For example, men in the upper occupational categories were most likely to perceive gains from their illness and to view life more positively as a result of their heart disease. (5) In general, other social status and demographic characteristics of the heart patients did not seem to be of predictive value in regard to Year 8 status variables. (6) Controlling for illness level did not substantially alter the findings on antecedents of outcome which emerged for the total study population. (7) Examination of selected pre-illness items concerning subjective stress and morale showed results congruent with those for the Year 1 to Year 8 measures. Thus, these traits before the illness were related to later variables indicating symptom level, emotional stress, and morale.

We examined patients' responses at Week 7 concerning their psychological characteristics prior to the first heart attack, using factor analysis. Those men who were characterized as high on the "emotional lability" factor before their illness, were most likely to report depressive reaction, subjective stress, frequent symptoms, low satisfaction with life, and a "work career affected by illness" 8 years later. When controls for severity of illness were introduced, pre-illness emotional lability linked to morale measures only for men without recent hospitalization. It was suggested that, because these men had not recently been ill, these earlier psychological characteristics might have been more prominent in determining general morale after 8 years than the fact of physical illness itself.

Within the context of the "armory of resources," the findings reported in this chapter point to particular current and antecedent factors which served as supports to the heart patients and enabled them to cope more constructively with their illness over the long term. Such resources include psychological characteristics of the patient reflecting ego strength and emotional stability. They include also occupational status before the illness, early morale and emotional response to the heart attack, and relative good health and recovery after the first heart attack. Several current variables, such as measures of interpersonal support and social participation, emerged as concomitants of more favorable outcome at Year 8.

We shall consider the implications of these findings in Chapter 9.

Notes

1. The complete list of symptoms was as follows: getting tired easily, chest pain, breathlessness, feeling heart is pounding or skipping a beat, swelling of the feet or ankles, sleeplessness, restlessness or nervousness, upset stomach, headaches, general aches and pains, loss of appetite, hands or feet shaking, spells of dizziness, fainting spells, cold sweats, pains from arthritis, and crying spells.

2. The four subjective stress items were as follows: (1) At the end of the day I am completely exhausted mentally and physically; (2) There is a great amount of nervous strain connected with my daily activities; (3) My daily activities are extremely trying and stressful; and (4) In general I am unusually tense and nervous. The total scale score was the sum of all the individual item weights and ranged from 4 to 16. Scores on the subjective stress scale are, therefore, inversely related to level of subjective stress, i.e., a low score represents high stress, while a high score symbolizes the absence of high stress. The procedure follows the original scoring method (Reeder *et al.*, 1973). The population was divided into terciles by the following method. A score of 10 and under was labeled "high," 11 through 14 was considered to be "medium," and 15 and over equaled "low."

3. The 2-year period was selected in part on conceptual grounds, in part on the basis of practical need to assure sufficient numbers in cells for analysis. A period of 1 year would have enabled the examination of those acutely ill most recently. However, in terms of initial comparisons between results of the 1-year period and the 2-year period, it was seen that results on statistical tests would not be significantly different on the whole. Therefore, in the interest of maximizing numbers in cells for analysis, the 2-year cut-off period was chosen. Much the same rationale formed the basis for the decision not to limit the hospitalization criterion to hospitalizations

for heart disease only. Rather, the hospitalized group includes men who reported hospitalization for any cause during the 2 years previous to the Year 8 interview.

4. As we indicated in Note 4 of Chapter 1, the chi-square test and the gamma correlation are our principal statistical tools. Level of significance has been set at .05.

Since this is an exploratory study, we consider it desirable to report findings that are in the direction of significance, but do not meet the formal criteria. Hence, we also report on findings at the .10 and .20 levels if they form a consistent pattern that might deserve future follow-up by other investigators. Such results are noted in the text as being in the direction of significance and suggestive of trends.

5. The following antecedent variables showed no pattern of association with patient status at Year 8: pre-illness family income, Year 1 valuation of religion, Year 1 frequency of lifting heavy weights at work, Week 7 physician assessment, presence of a confidant pre-illness, and self-description of "easily depressed" pre-illness.

6. For those men who had suffered recent hospitalization, however, a high score on pre-illness "emotional lability" was associated with more frequent reports of symptoms at Year 8. This was not the case for men not recently hospitalized.

Chapter 9

SUMMARY AND IMPLICATIONS

INTRODUCTION

In this chapter, we summarize our major approaches and findings and integrate some of the main conclusions and recommendations which emerge from our study. We propose some applications and policy recommendations for patient management, the planning of services, and the designation of target populations for special support.

This report builds upon the materials of our previous baseline study of heart patients in Greater Boston. In our earlier research we asked: what happens to men who have been living normal lives and who then experience a first life-threatening episode of major illness? What is the nature of their subsequent experience in principal areas of their lives? What factors most influence their adjustments after a limited period of time, such as 1 year? In this follow-up study after 8 years, we consider a series of similar issues. Meanwhile, however, the factors operating have developed new complexity, involving changes associated with aging, additional illnesses, the occurrence of other influential life events, and trends in the sociocultural environment.

THE ARMORY OF RESOURCES: PHYSICAL, PSYCHOLOGICAL, SOCIAL, AND COMMUNITY SUPPORTS

In pursuing our research questions, we have focused on man as a coping creature who possesses an array of resources and capacities consisting of personal, social, institutional, organizational, and community elements, which enable him to deal with life contingencies. The resources constitute an armory upon which the individual can draw.

We have operationalized the concept of armory of resources in terms of several principal areas, designating various measures for each. Some illustrations are:

1. *Physical resources:* measures of patients' health status, including physician assessments; patients' self-reports on activity and physical capacity; and items of record such as survival and rehospitalization data.

2. *Psychological resources:* morale, presence or absence of depressive reaction to the illness, various psychological characteristics indicative of emotional status and lability.

3. *Social supports:* family structure; marital status, marital integration; presence of wife as confidant; informal social participation; club memberships; aid and assistance received from family, neighbors, friends; church attendance and the personal meaning of religion.

4. *Community and professional supports:* physician services; continuity of the doctor-patient relationship; use of agencies, institutions, and other professionals, such as employment agencies, rehabilitation units; use of government programs, and cash benefits.

The classification is by no means intended as a rigid one. The nature of the resources is such that a particular item, such as a social support, may have psychological and community aspects as well. This framework served as a guide to our selection of operational measures, facilitating our exploration of the relative influence of resource variables upon long-term outcome.

With this population of men with heart disease, we sought to document and describe some aspects of their life experience and use of supports in each of the major resource areas. We wished also to explore the long-term illness careers of men who differed in age, social status characteristics, psychological characteristics, and medical prognosis. In a sense, the framework is simple, but it permits a multifaceted approach to a complex set of problems involving the human experience and life with illness.

Our approach rests on a view of illness as an event occurring within a complex social and cultural context, one in which there are many interrelations between the various subsystems in which a patient is involved. These subsystems present to the patient a broad range of potential resources upon which he can draw. The patient in turn exerts influences upon these systems. Thus, a family may provide a support during illness; the sick person, in turn, influences the activities and response of the family, affecting its capacity and willingness to provide support.

In recent years, much research interest has turned to the ways in which social supports and social networks affect the capacity of persons to cope with illness and with other events in their lives. But, important as these social supports and networks may be, they are but one aspect of the total armamentarium. Hence, in our efforts here to document the long-term experience of heart patients, we have chosen a holistic approach to give emphasis to the broad range of potential resources which may be called upon. Thus, along with social supports, we consider other diverse aspects of the physical, psychological, social, and community resources as key elements for reference and exploration. Although we may discuss the various resources and supports individually, we keep in mind, of course, that they actually operate in combination as they enable individuals to cope.

THE STUDY POPULATION: AN 8-YEAR PERSPECTIVE

Because of the special nature of the original selection criteria, the men in our base-line study were clearly not typical heart patients. In fact, they were an elite group in many respects. They survived the critical first days after their heart attacks, and left the hospital after an uncomplicated course of recovery. As men without previous major illness, they were, on the whole, persons with relatively favorable medical prognoses. As men pursuing a full range of activities before the heart attack, they had much to live for.

In this long-term follow-up study, that same population now has a somewhat different profile. The focus of our present research effort begins at a point 1 year after a first heart attack. At the 1-year stage, all the patients had medical histories of progressive coronary artery disease. Hence, the study population had become more similar to the general population of heart patients with histories of hospitalization for myocardial infarction.

Nevertheless, after 8 years, the study population maintains many of its other special characteristics. Nearly all the patients in our study live in a metropolitan area of the Northeast United States. They live in a social and cultural climate distinctive for its historic traditions and emotional tone. The area is noted for its concentration of medical facilities and educational institutions. It shares with other American metropolitan areas such traits as urban occupations, rapid communication, rapid transportation, and a heterogeneous ethnic population. The patients had available to them, therefore, a broad range of resources, services, and facilities.

THE APPROACH TO LONG-TERM OUTCOME: EXAMINATION OF MULTIPLE STATUSES

One of the primary questions toward which this research was directed concerned the patterns of long-term outcome and variables which might be considered as possible predictors of these. Through our prospective approach we collected data which might bear on these issues, at least in an exploratory way. As we explained in Chapter 8, procedures in measuring outcome were designed to minimize value judgments in regard to adjustment or adaptation. Thus, we measured outcome by use of the notion of statuses, comparing position or status on a series of variables at different points in time. These were classified into *primary* and *secondary status index* variables, each set providing a somewhat differing perspective on outcome.

We have avoided a reductionist approach which would involve summation of all the ratings into a single index score, although this might be useful for some purposes. Instead, we followed the rationale that in looking at the total pattern of statuses in a study which is mainly exploratory and descriptive, it is necessary to examine each individual part. One can make no assumptions *a priori* that one variable is related to another. A patient may be employed but have low morale. A patient may have disabling symptoms but remain employed, even working long hours despite the symptoms. Hence, in line with our multi-dimensional model of the recovery and rehabilitation process, we have generally preferred to examine separately these subparts or statuses in various areas of the lives of the patients. At the present stage in development of knowledge in this area, the approach promotes a balanced view of the complex subparts which comprise the patient's career.

Our principal findings in regard to outcome can be summarized in two parts: mortality-morbidity aspects and social-psychological issues.

Long-Term Outcome: A Brief Review

Mortality-Morbidity

The long-term "medical fate" of the patients over the course of 8 years appeared to be best explained by their previous physical status. Those who were most ill at the beginning of the study did not fare as well as those who were less ill. This finding was consistently reproduced when we employed differing health status measures, including assessments by the physicians, self-ratings of symptoms by the patients, and the record of rehospitalizations during the first year.

Although we employed various perspectives and methods of statistical analysis in examining the data, in general we were not able to explain rehospitalizations and mortality from heart disease by the social, demographic, or psychological characteristics of the patients, as measured in this study. Certain indicators of emotional status at Year 1, such as depressive reaction to the illness, were associated with medical outcome, but these characteristics may be interpreted as part of the total syndrome of response to cardiovascular disease.

The progressive and chronic nature of the disease is also reflected in the record of subsequent rehospitalizations for heart disease within a considerable segment of the study population. Over the course of the years it was heart disease which was the principal cause of death. In a sense, that first heart attack might be seen as a "predictor" of eventual cause of death for most of the men. Such data are consistent, of course, with the experience of insurance companies and with the actuarial estimates which guide their policy.

There was a conspicuous exception to our lack of positive findings in regard to health outcome and social, psychological, and demographic traits of the patients. Our data showed significantly higher mortality from subsequent heart attacks among semiskilled and unskilled men and low-income men during the study period. At the least, such a finding deserves further scrutiny and raises some serious questions as to why such differential patterns of death should occur. We suggested possible explanations in Chapter 2.

Social-Psychological

A second set of findings suggests that social and psychological statuses at 8 years were generally not explained by the antecedent physical measures from the first year. Severity of illness and other indicators of physical condition at Year 1 were less important as antecedents of social and psychological status at Year 8 than were previous indicators of emotional status, morale, social integration, and work involvement. For example, among these heart patients, decline in social participation at Year 8 was not simply attributable to failing physical capacity and increasing symptoms.

Perhaps the clearest message in the data is the potential value of early social and psychological variables as predictors of later social and emotional statuses. Thus, the men who reported high morale and satisfaction with life at Year 1 were the most likely to report high morale and life satisfaction 7 years later. Those who enjoyed social integration and personal and family supports in the base-line study reported the same life circumstances at Year 8. Data on emotional lability, moodiness, and tendency for depressive reaction early in the study were useful for predicting similar emotional states at Year 8.

We also found a pattern of current correlates of outcome measures or statuses at Year 8. The picture is one of apparent high internal consistency. The men with highest morale and life satisfaction were those who concurrently reported a low number of symptoms, presence of a confidant, lack of depressive reaction, and related characteristics. While these variables are derived from different areas of the lives of patients, each may be tapping the more general dimension of "well-being."

Such statistical findings are easily open to misinterpretation, and in line with our conservative approach, we wish to offer some words of caution regarding generalization. For example, because of statistical relationships between level of symptoms and positive morale, one might be led erroneously to assume causality in some degree rather than a corelationship. The fact that positive morale is found among some persons with low symptoms should not be interpreted as an indication that favorable psychological state leads to a reduction in severity of heart disease. The presence of a confidant was also negatively associated with level of symptoms, but this does not imply that patients have few symptoms because they have a confidant. In other words, this study cannot in any way imply from its available data that the long-term arteriosclerotic process is alterable by high positive morale or by having someone to talk to. It would be improper to interpret such data on coassociation in terms of causality, even though the interpretations may be consistent with psychogenic theories of etiology of illness.

In general, findings of this follow-up study show a continuity with those of our base-line research covering the year after the first heart attack (Croog & Levine, 1977). Although numerous events and circumstances had intervened in the period between Year 1 and Year 8, the principal basic "predictors" at Year 8 remained similar to those found in the first year.

In sum, what do these data on outcomes in the medical and the sociopsychological areas tell us? It seems evident that long-term "physical fate" is most closely related to health status, i.e., level of impairment, which existed at the beginning of this prospective study.

But how the patients *deal* with their illness, how they come to terms with it, and with its implications for their lives appears to be related both to the kinds of persons they were early in the illness, and to the resources or supports which aid them. In general, those patients with many social supports and a high level of personal-social integration and life rewards at the time of their first heart attack seemed to be similarly characterized 8 years later.

AGE, AGING, AND HEART DISEASE

One feature of the study design was that it enabled us to collect data on patients at successive stages in the life cycle of the older adult. In the base-line study, we saw the men first when their average age was in the mid-50s. When we interviewed them again for this follow-up research, most were either approaching or at retirement age. At the time of Year 8, we were able to examine a population which was coping with the dual problems of aging and chronic illness.

In our exploration of age and aging in relation to heart disease, we followed several lines of interest, viewing age both as a characteristic of the cohort and as a specific variable in the analysis. Thus, one line of interest involved describing a cohort of heart patients at an advanced point in the life cycle, reporting on various features of their life problems, use of resources and services, and other matters we have already noted. Another was the relationship of age to such various elements as work, family, compliance with the medical regimen, and psychological characteristics. Here we examined age as a possible correlate of variation in social and psychological patterns in the context of heart disease. A third line of interest involved comparison between two cohorts in regard to areas of life adjustment. These two consisted of (1) an older group of men at Year 8, and (2) the younger cohort, consisting of the same men at an earlier age, at Week 7 or Year 1.

One principal finding was that age itself did not explain differential morbidity or mortality in our data. Nor was it a useful variable at Year 8 for differentiating the population on most of the items we examined.

Age did emerge as a correlate of some outcome variables, of course. As one might expect, among men of similar illness levels, the older men were most likely to retire. But here too, the pattern was not entirely age related, for there was a social class differential as well. Moreover, older men had a higher positive orientation toward compliance with the medical regimen than did the younger patients. They also used more physician services. For the most part, however, the older men did not differ significantly from the younger men on the principal outcome variables we examined at Year 8.

We also examined data on stability and change in social and psychological characteristics in relation to age. We analyzed responses to the same questions at differing periods, comparing base-line data with those of the follow-up study at Year 8. On the whole, few relationships between age and changes in response emerged. With a few exceptions, reports of behavior and beliefs at Year 8 did not differ significantly from those which the patients had given as younger men years earlier.

What does this all mean? Is there a message in the data with regard to the influence of age on adjustment to heart disease? The results must be viewed in perspective and with appropriate qualifications. In the first place, the lack of significant correlates of age at both stages may be due to the limited range of ages; a large percentage of the study population was concentrated within a 15-year age range. Further, this study did not include men in their 70s, 80s, or 90s. If the upper age limit of the study population had extended into age groups subject to problems of senility and of impairment due to aging, more age-related phenomena clearly would have emerged.

Given these qualifications, however, the findings have some positive features. They show, for example, that within the age span of the patients at Year 8, differences in age level appear to account for few observed variations in patterns. Morbidity, mortality, finances, self-rated psychological characteristics, morale, emotional lability, or support from family members and quasi-kin specifically were not age related. In the matters of work, finances, and retirement, the picture is somewhat more complex, for obvious reasons. If high proportions of older men retire, their financial circumstances will clearly differ from those of younger men.

These findings may have important ramifications for planning supportive and health services for patients at these points in the life cycle. If age is not a major differentiating factor, efforts at planning may perhaps be directed more economically to many problems without concern for age gradations, at least as far as this age-span group is concerned. Exceptions, of course, are in the areas of retirement planning and organizing supportive services required after retirement. But even here, because retirement can take place at any age, it is the retirement situation rather than the pure age variable itself which may have to be addressed.

In other words, in this population of heart patients, to be an older man and retired does not necessarily imply unique problems. In fact, for many such men, the life satisfactions and personal rewards were greater than for the younger men.

USE OF RESOURCES AND PATTERNS OF SOCIAL SUPPORTS

In line with our principal aims for this research, we examined a series of differing types of resources and supports in regard to their role in the lives of the heart patients. We turn now to a brief review of findings.

The Physician as Resource

The Doctor-Patient Relationship. As one might expect in a study of patients with chronic illness in the United States, the physician is a key figure in the long-term care and guidance of the heart patients in our research. The experience of the heart patients with their physicians bears special note, given the prevalence of criticism of the medical profession in this country and the misgivings about the fate of the doctor-patient relationship.

Over the period of the study since Year 1, the majority of patients continued to see the same physician in connection with their illness. Three-fourths of the patients with some college, about two-thirds of high school graduates, and over half of those who did not graduate from high school continued their treatment with the same physician as at Year 1. This pattern occurred despite such factors as the retirement or death of some of the original physicians, the geographical mobility of patients, the greater use of clinic services by patients in the lower socioeconomic levels, and the spread of group medical practice.

In our first book we reported that during the year after the first heart attack, considerable proportions of patients expressed satisfaction with their physicians and indicated their intention to continue under the same doctor's care. The Year 8 data clearly demonstrate the fulfillment of these intentions, and they show that, in the main, patients were satisfied with the care they received. The actual behavior of these patients over many years provides a convincing demonstration of their feelings of approval, basic trust, and loyalty toward their doctors.

We found no differences in volume of use of physician services among men of differing educational levels or socioeconomic status. This finding is also consistent with other Year 8 data on orientation to compliance with the medical regimen. It should be noted, however, that these results are not congruent with the findings of other studies. Other researchers have reported that the more educated populations are more frequent users of physician services, attributing this in part to their presumed interest in prevention and in having continuing medical supervision (Aday & Eichhorn, 1972).

Physicians and Compliance with the Medical Regimen

At 8 years after their first heart attack, nearly all the patients (over 90%) reported having been given instructions for a current medical regimen by their physicians. The patients varied in their level of health, of course, and in the specific regimen prescribed.

On many items of physician advice, half or more of the patients who received such advice reported partial or total noncompliance. Given that these particular data derive from patient reports rather than objective measures, it appears highly likely that actual compliance behavior was even less than many patients indicated.

When we sought predictors of positive compliance orientation, our findings resembled those which have been reported in numerous other studies. The data showed no consistent patterns of relationship between compliance with the medical regimen and social, psychological, and demographic variables. Along with this general pattern, there were several interesting findings of a more limited nature.

First, the item of advice which elicited the highest positive compliance orientation was "medications." This is possibly due to the fact that patients find instructions on medication most easy to comply with. Taking medications is a repetitive, clearly defined, and comparatively simple task. Further, evidence of therapeutic benefit can be convincing, in contrast to other physician advice in which the benefits may be less clear-cut.

Second, in contrast to our own findings during Year 1, and unlike other research concerned with compliance, we found that age was related in a positive way to compliance orientation. Third, it appeared that the best predictor of compliance orientation at Year 8 was an earlier favorable compliance orientation at Week 7 and Year 1. In other terms, once again a general principle of human behavior was apparently reaffirmed: that one of the best predictors of future performance is past performance.

Some of our most striking findings resulted from our longitudinal examination of smoking patterns and compliance with physician advice. The data revealed a consistent and persisting reduction after the first heart attack in number of cigarettes smoked. The initial decline in smoking evident in the first year was still apparent in the patient population at Year 8. Although this decline in the heart patient group is consistent with the national secular trend, it is clearly a far more dramatic one. How could this finding emerge given the usual reports of difficulty in effecting long-term changes in health behavior? We have suggested that heart disease—as a lethal, unpredictable illness—constitutes an especially potent stimulus. After hospitalization for myocardial infarction, heart patients are well aware of its power and consequences. Patients may eventually come to realize that there is no "negotiation with fate," that their survival is clearly at stake, that they must adhere to the medical regimen in regard to smoking.

Judging from data on both medications and smoking reduction, further, it appears that patients may tend to comply on those advice items which seem to be most clear-cut in their benefits. But they are less inclined to follow the regimen on items which have only a long-term or less certain advantage. In all of this, as we have seen, the role of the physician as a continuing support and guide is a paramount one in the armory of resources of patients.

The Community and Society: Services as Resources

At the time of this research, the communities of Greater Boston and Worcester were rich in health care, rehabilitative, and social service organizations. However, the evidence shows minimal use of such community resources by the patient population during both the base-line and follow-up study periods.

Lacking direct information on the reasons for low utilization during Year 1, one might easily conclude at that time that the findings were not surprising. After all, most patients had remained reasonably well during the year, and at that stage in their illness careers, perhaps the services were mainly inappropriate, not relevant, or simply not needed.

At Year 8 it was possible to look back on patterns of utilization of agency and professional services once again, this time from a different standpoint. Many in the study population had by now experienced recurrent episodes of illness and additional rehospitalizations. The volume and scope of problems associated with illness and with aging had expanded. Yet as we have seen, the earlier pattern of minimal use of services was still evident, both within the year prior to the Year 8 interview and over the 7 years between Year 1 and Year 8. Given the increase in apparent "need" among many patients, this low usage of services is a particularly notable finding.

The findings are especially interesting in view of the missions of some of the professionals and agencies who were not utilized. For example, although a substantial proportion of the patients had been rehospitalized and suffered varying degrees of disability, few men reported use of services of the Visiting Nurses Association. Only five men reported contact with a Cardiac Rehabilitation Unit in the years between Year 1 and Year 8. Not many turned to the clergy to discuss problems and concerns stemming from their illness. While the percentages reporting use of particular services may be understated because of problems of recall or other factors, it seems clear that actual utilization of the community resources was still relatively low.

Work and Finances

At 8 years after the first heart attack, the work status of the patient population was more varied than in the base-line study. Before the initial illness, nearly all the men had been employed (Croog & Levine, 1977). By the end of Year 1, furthermore, nearly all were back at work or were seeking employment.

By Year 8, nearly one-third of the surviving group had left the work force or had reduced their work load to part time. Of course, by now most of these men had already reached or were approaching the age at which they would ordinarily retire. But the influence of illness was often of considerable importance in affecting employment and retirement decisions. Among those who were no longer full-time workers, nearly three-quarters cited their health as a major factor in the decision to retire or to cut back on their working days.

One factor bearing on the retirement decision was the widespread belief among the men that their work had been a risk to their health. Fully three-quarters of the employed men at Year 8 stated the view that emotional tension and/or physical exertion on the job had been a factor in the etiology of their most recent heart attack. A similar proportion had expressed the same view in the base-line study (Croog & Levine, 1977). However, many of the men who regarded their work as a cause of their heart attacks remained employed. In effect, they were returning daily to work situations which they perceived as threatening to their health and lives.

Along with adding to the stress levels of the workers, these beliefs can also influence the attitudes of employers toward employees with heart disease. Men with a history of heart disease, subject to recurrence of the acute phase and believing that work contributed to their heart attack, represent high risk from the perspective of an employer. Because of their health history, such men may be particularly vulnerable for impairment, disability, and death from heart disease. And their beliefs make them more likely than other workers to make legal claims on the basis of dangers to their health in the work place. Such considerations may serve to inhibit the development of appropriate cardiac programs in industry.

Many of the men who remained employed continued to work in a manner which they believed might harm their health. For example, high proportions of executives and professionals who cited work tension as a factor in the etiology of their heart attacks continued to work 50 to 70 hours per week. This same occupational group, it should be noted, also reported the most subjective work stress at various points in our longitudinal study.

These findings underline the relative difficulty of inducing changes in work behavior for reasons of health. When a man continues to work in a way he believes may harm him, there are no simple ways to help him to reduce his efforts. There are potent social, psychological, and economic factors which underlie decisions by men to work long hours, even when they believe work stresses may induce another heart attack.

At Year 8 most patients, both currently employed and retired, recalled experiencing few or no problems at work as a result of their heart conditions. However, a substantial minority did so. Within individual occupational groups their number ranged from one-quarter to one-third of the patients.

Professional men and executives, in particular, felt that their illness had had negative effects on their promotion or long-term advancement. Higher proportions of white-collar than blue-collar workers reported negative effects on relations with their employers. It is interesting to note that in the base-line study the blue-collar and semiskilled men made more pessimistic predictions about the long-term effects of illness on promotion and advancement than did the executives and professionals. But the reported experience of the surviving cohort 8 years later was quite different, and the heart condition had turned out to be far more of a handicap for the executives and professionals than they had envisioned earlier.

On the whole, out-of-pocket costs of illness and illness-related financial issues in general seemed less troubling at Year 8 than in the first year. An important factor, of course, is that, in contrast to Year 1, only a part of the population at Year 8 had recently experienced recurrence of the acute phase of the illness and hospitalization.

Only a small proportion of men in the work force at Year 8 indicated that illness during the previous year had led to loss of income. Even when we looked only at those employed men who had been rehospitalized in the 12 months prior to the Year 8 interview, the pattern was the same. In contrast, in the base-line study a considerable proportion of the employed patients, particularly blue-collar men, reported income loss due to the first heart attack.

Over the years of the study, few wives were forced to obtain employment as a result of illness of their husbands. Many of the patients' wives were already employed when the study began, and those women who subsequently took jobs did so mainly for reasons other than financial stresses brought on by the illness.

Reported out-of-pocket expenditures for medicines, physicians' bills, and other medical care were relatively low at Year 8. This was due, in part, to the protection afforded by Medicare and by other forms of hospital and medical insurance. In general, illness-related costs and finances were not perceived as the most critical issues by the patient population. When asked about their biggest concerns for the future, only one-fifth of the patients at Year 8 mentioned finances.

There are several possible explanations for this finding. One is that compared to basic issues of health and sheer survival, problems of finances seemed relatively less critical to this group of heart patients. We can hypothesize also that the nature of the interview question obscured the true incidence of perception of finances and money as major problems. Still another explanation is that at this point in the lives of the patients, problems of money and finances were so pervasive that they were indeed unremarkable—part of the conditions of normal life after 8 years of chronic illness.[1]

In connection with this issue of perception of problems, studies of attitudes of elderly persons toward their health may have relevance. These studies have shown that older people tend more to take illness for granted, perceiving their health as something less than perfect well-being, a condition including symptoms with which they must live. Perhaps a similar perspective influenced the responses of patients about financial matters. Having many concerns involving money might be so common-place that it was regarded as not worthy of mention as a principal, salient problem.

Work Stresses and Heart Disease

One of our findings raises questions that may be resolved only by further research. While the semiskilled and unskilled workers suffered conspicuously higher mortality rates from heart disease than other heart patients by Year 8, there is no evidence in our study that this can be attributed to differential emotional stress at work. It will be recalled that at Year 8, the lower occupational groups of heart patients in fact reported experiencing less emotional stress at work in comparison to other groups. Further, as we saw in Chapter 2, work stresses before the first heart attack and at Year 1 did not appear to be risk factors in mortality and/or rehospitalizations for heart disease during the years of the follow-up study.

Our findings raise questions, but hardly resolve the issue of the relationship between work stress and mortality. It must be emphasized, first of all, that our study does not focus on etiology, but on subsequent experience of patients who already have suffered a primary myocardial infarction. However, in our previous study of heart patients at Year 1, manual workers reported more difficulties in returning to work, and a greater proportion of this group, as compared with other occupational categories, sought to modify the requirements of the job because of their illness. Still, at Year 1 as well as at Year 8, a smaller proportion of manual workers reported emotional stress at work, in comparison with white-collar workers, executives, and professionals.

The literature is not always consistent on the relationship between stress and heart disease. In one of the most thorough reviews of the role of social and psychological factors in the etiology of heart disease, Jenkins (1976) drew attention to incon-sistencies in the findings. He posited, however, that in the early stages of industrialization the higher status workers were subject to more overall stress and accordingly experienced more heart disease. In later stages of economic development, the situation is allegedly reversed, Jenkins suggests, with the manual labor populations presumably exposed to greater stress and, accordingly, more subject to heart disease and other illnesses.

It is likely then that the negative effects of lower occupational status are felt pervasively in areas of life other than work—in the inequities in daily living, in the more exacting and demanding pressures of life, in having one's psychic, physical, and social resources exhausted over a lifetime, so that one is more vulnerable when a second or third heart attack is experienced. Another explanation may be that social status is associated with a style of life—eating, smoking, sleeping, and other habits or activities— which may account for the differential mortality among the various occupational groups. Finally, whether or not emotional stress on the job does in fact play a role in the onset of the first heart attack, it is also possible that after the first attack is experienced, such stress may play only a minor role, or its effects may be overridden by other factors. Whatever the explanation, the strikingly high mortality rate among the lowest occupational groups merits further study and deliberation.

Cash Benefit Programs and Finances

Social Security was the most utilized cash benefit program, as might be expected with an aging population. Social Security disability insurance programs, however, apply to men of any age. As we have seen, Social Security made payments for disability benefits to this population in higher proportion than did private insurance companies. Worker's Compensation and welfare programs provided income to relatively few heart patients during the 12 months prior to the Year 8 interview.

One feature of the Social Security data was the differing pattern among men of varying educational level. The least educated men applied in the highest proportions for some type of Social Security benefit. They also outranked men of other educational levels in receipt of Social Security disability benefits during the previous year.

As we might anticipate, those men with multiple rehospitalizations were more likely than others to receive Social Security disability payments. And, again as one might expect, most of the patients receiving Social Security benefits noted the inadequacy of payments as supplements to their income.

The Family as Resource

In the base-line study, the key role of the family as a source of aid and support was clearly evident. In fact, the strong support provided the patients by close relatives contradicted many portrayals in the professional literature and the media about the decline of the extended family and the shifting of its functions to the larger society. In the study of Year 1 we reported also on the important role of non-kin groups such as friends and neighbors in providing support and we suggested that they were functioning as quasi-family.

Now, at Year 8, the men and their families were older and various age-related circumstances had occurred. The base-line study did not examine the supportive role of children because of difficulties presented by their widely varying ages. Some were too young to be realistically considered in relation to the support they might provide. But now, at Year 8, in most of the families the children were adults or in late adolescence. Meanwhile, a large proportion of patients had retired, and new family relationships were operative. Finally, patients' needs were more varied now, given their differing life circumstances and health levels.

Even so, essentially the same findings emerged at Year 8 as at the earlier stages. Kin and quasi-kin groups continued to be perceived as approximately equal in importance to the patients as resources. A particular exception is in the high citation of children. In their elder years, those heart patients with mature children saw them as significantly more important resources than any other relatives, friends, or neighbors.

It might be assumed that the amount of aid patients received varied with their objective "need" or severity of illness at Year 8. We found, however, that support and resources provided by family members was part of a broader social matrix of interaction, involving kin and non-kin. In brief, those who received aid or support from one source were also likely to report it from others. We observed a similar finding in the base-line study of the first year as well. The data perhaps point up once again the distinctive and sustained problems of the socially isolated, or less socially integrated individuals.

These data on supports from family and non-kin should be evaluated in relation to the use of other types of resources. Obviously, the physician stands alone as a technical resource, and family and non-kin groups for the most part do not duplicate physicians' services. But more striking is the fact that the patients made minimal use of other professionals and formal services in the community, while reporting aid and assistance from children, other kin, and non-kin persons. In terms of moral support, services, and financial aid, it would appear that family and quasi-family in general played a more important role than the agencies of the community. This finding, as we have noted, is not congruent with many theories about the increasing assumption of former family functions by the larger community. The results, of course, obviously pertain only to this study population—a group characterized by chronic illness—and they cannot be generalized to populations in other circumstances.

Psychological Characteristics: An 8-Year Perspective

The exact role of personality factors in recovery and rehabilitation after a heart attack persists as an important and still controversial issue. In the course of this study, we were able to carry out some exploratory analyses of aspects of psychological status of the heart patients. By asking many of the same questions in interviews over the course of 8 years, we gained a longitudinal perspective which has rarely been feasible in research on the psychological status of cardiac populations.

One principal finding was that the self-rated psychological characteristics were very stable over the period of the study, despite numerous intervening events and processes, such as aging, additional illness, changing life circumstances, and perhaps even conscious efforts to change aspects of personality. It is often hypothesized that serious illness may alter personality considerably, but in the case of the psychological self-ratings which we examined, the data lend little support to the hypothesis. Instead, the findings were more consistent with classical psychological theories that posit the basic stability of the ego and of self-image, particularly in the adult.

Thus, men who were hard driving and ambitious before the first heart attack appeared, in general, to still possess these same characteristics at Year 8. Even though many of these men believed that stress and tension were important factors in the etiology of their illness, there is little evidence that these men changed in their personality orientation, at least in terms of the measures employed in this study. For example, those men who reported disturbances of mood occurring before the first infarction—emotional lability, moodiness, tendency toward depressive reaction—were likely to describe themselves the same way at Year 8. Men who were initially less emotionally labile and reported less depressive reaction, tended to remain that way over time. While ours is not a formal "predictive" study, these data suggest that early knowledge of psychological self-ratings may predict later psychological characteristics, despite the press of intervening events and illness experiences.

In the literature of psychosomatic medicine, numerous formulations characterize types of personality which are prone to develop particular illnesses. In the case of this heart patient population—all of whom had manifest disease with at least one acute phase—it was possible to explore at least some principal ways in which the patients see themselves. Over many decades the coronary personality has been described as a distinctive type, often labeled in part as hard driving, ambitious, and easily angered. In more recent years, earlier formulations have been reinforced through evidence pointing to the Type A "coronary-prone behavior pattern," as described by Friedman, Rosenman, Jenkins, and others. In the heart patient study population, "classic" coronary psychological characteristics did not appear as strong or pervasive as we might have predicted on the basis of the theoretical literature, although some men did exhibit such characteristics.

A persisting question in studies of heart patients is whether recurrences of heart attacks are related to personality orientation. Do men who are hard driving, ambitious, and aggressive have a greater probability of recurrence? When we examined self-rated characteristics and subsequent recurrence of heart attacks in the heart patients, no significant relationships were found. Others using the Structured Interview and Jenkins "Type A" Scale have found some suggestive relationships between the Type A "coronary-prone behavior pattern" and recurrence (Friedman, 1979; Jenkins, Zyzanski, & Rosenman, 1976; Kenigsberg et al., 1974).

One apparent exception to our findings on psychological status and recurrence is the association between depressive reaction and subsequent recurrence and death. Patients who described themselves as depressed over their illness at Year 1 had a higher probability of subsequent cardiac events. By knowing who was depressed early in response to the illness, it could thus be possible to predict probability of subsequent outcomes.

The data are consistent on the whole with the reactive aspects implicit in the term "depressive reaction." Those men who were depressed over the illness were also likely to be those with the greatest impairment and poorest prognostic ratings by their physicians. Hence, we can hypothesize that they experienced recurrences because they were initially the sickest and their depressive reaction was part of the pattern of symptoms associated with severe illness. More simply, we can suggest that the sickest men had more reason to be depressed and, in fact, had a higher proportion of recurrences than the men who did not report depressive reactions.

In considering these explanations, of course, we cannot dismiss alternative hypotheses, such as those holding that psychological factors—perhaps the depressive reaction itself—had an etiological influence upon recurrence. In any case we must emphasize that evaluation of the meaning of such findings must await more fine-grained analysis partialling out the effects of a broad series of other variables, including physiological, biochemical, and behavioral measures.

Emotional Burdens of Heart Disease: Implications From the Data

The emotional concomitants of chronic illness are well known to clinicians who treat heart patients, and they appear as persisting issues in our data. In many patients, depressive reaction, subjective stress and tension, and anxiety are evident over the course of 8 years. They were expressed in part in symptoms of sleeplessness, nervousness, digestive disorders, as well as in disturbances of mood and emotional lability. For many patients, such symptoms of emotional distress were not experienced as single, limited episodes. As we have seen, those who reported symptoms of depressive reaction, mood disturbances, and emotional lability early in the illness were also likely to report them years later.

To be a person with heart disease means living not only with the physical illness, but also with its emotional burdens. They can be implied only in a limited way by the written word: The awareness of the possibility of unpredictable, sudden death. The recognition that the pain and acute illness of previous heart attacks can occur again. The presence, in many patients, of chest pain, shortness of breath, and the inability to walk for even moderate distances without symptoms. The need to take multiple medications daily, with each occasion serving as a reminder of the underlying condition and threat. Living with the occasional or persisting side effects of medications, including such symptoms as dizziness or vertigo, digestive disturbances, depression, reduced energy level, reduced sex drive, and possible impotence. The continued reminder of one's own mortality and the unpredictability of life from one moment to another.

Moreover, the illness and its emotional concomitants also touch others with whom the patient associates—his family, friends, and people at the work place. In regard to the family, for example, we reported how the illness raised the level of anxiety and concern among wives and children, pointing up some variations in degree of these responses among families. We also pointed up many ways in which wives and other family members provided important nurturance and support for the heart patient over the years.

But we must also note that in some families there was evidence of deeper and more disturbing disruptions associated with the illness. In considering the etiology of their heart attacks, relatively high proportions of men cited conflicts with wives and with children as contributing factors. In our first study, furthermore, we reported that numerous wives, too, cited marital conflict as a contributing cause of the heart attack in their husbands.

How does living with such beliefs affect the quality of family life? In what ways does the husband express recrimination and accusation? What are the effects of defensive response and of feelings of guilt on the part of wives? And what effects do such tensions in the marital relationship have upon the illness of the patient and his long-term course of recovery? Such questions have particular relevance for heart disease because of the well-known laboratory evidence of cardiovascular response to psychological stressors as well as clinical evidence of the effects of emotional shock upon the heart.

All the patients in this study were confronted with the problem of emotional adjustment to the illness, and some reached happier resolutions than others. We know that for some, the emotional burdens of the illness proved particularly heavy. The size of this group cannot be determined precisely. Use of the survey research method undoubtedly obscured the true level of emotional malaise and distress in this population. In regard to the issues of greatest emotional sensitivity, some patients unquestionably gave socially acceptable responses rather than reveal their deeper feelings. In some instances, it is probable that the mechanism of denial was operative, and patients were thus unable to recognize or verbalize the deep emotional distress which they were experiencing.

The point here is that it is likely that the survey research data tend to understate the prevalence of emotional problems in the study population. Problems of measurement, fluctuations in emotional distress over time, and issues of definition all lead us to caution about underestimating the psychological sequelae of the illness in the heart patient group. This issue is of some consequence here insofar as it reflects upon the possible need for services or for supportive intervention in the course of medical treatment and rehabilitation. Medical care survey data, as reported by physicians, show that in a recent year in two-thirds of office visits by heart patients, contact with the doctor lasted 15 minutes or less (National Center for Health Statistics, 1978). In the office of the physician, as in the survey research interview, the lack of expression of problems of emotional adjustment during brief contact does not imply their absence, and it does not reduce the desirability of considering such factors in planning the medical regimen.

Conclusions and Recommendations

We have considered a broad range of social, psychological, economic, and situational factors in the long-term careers of the heart patients. The patient's "armory of resources" provided us with a guiding framework to examine his various types of personal, social, community, and societal supports. Through this procedure, we have been able to review and describe some problems and outcomes which emerged over the course of 8 years, noting how these applied to patients with varying social, psychological, and health-level characteristics.

This approach, as we have seen, has enabled us to examine some of the complex elements which influence how the long-term outcomes of heart disease are determined. In some ways the data in this report have an optimistic message. For among the several hundred men in the original study group, many lived in happy circumstances throughout the full period covered by our research. Moreover, most of the patients continued to participate in varied phases of daily living and to perform their major social roles.

After a period of 8 years, they have incorporated their heart condition along with other problems into the pattern of their daily lives. It is a testimony to people's remarkable ability to adapt to their burdens when there are stable anchors in their lives and continuity in their fundamental social relationships.

Despite these encouraging findings, our study also underlines the fact that our patients are suffering from a disease which is chronic and unremitting in many ways. While the survival rate is reassuring, the majority of such patients at some time will experience a variety of serious physical as well as emotional symptoms. Further, as we reported, about half suffered one or more recurrences of their heart attacks during the study period, and half of these died.

Our findings suggest that we can be fairly effective in *predicting* which patients are most likely to experience specific types of problems. The advantage of the longitudinal approach which we have taken is that we have been able to ascertain what features at the onset of the illness persist almost a decade later, as well as how factors manifest at the beginning may help predict other problems subsequently. First, those patients who are more severely ill at Week 7 are most likely to have health problems at Year 8. Accordingly, physicians should devote particular attention to these patients, maintain close contact with them, and be readily available to them.

Second, a brief psychological profile should be obtained on each heart patient at an early stage which may be useful in predicting subsequent psychological and emotional problems. It may not be the specific task of the doctor to do much about this, but it is his responsibility to make sure that something is done.

Considering emotional health at 8 years as an outcome, certain variables from the earlier period appeared to be useful predictors of target populations, at least on initial scrutiny. For example, persons with depressive reactions in the base-line study were more likely to report depressive reactions during the follow-up period. As the depressive reaction may have been part of the total syndrome of continuing cardiovascular illness, these data may simply be showing in another way that serious cardiovascular disease is a progressive, long-term process. However, we should also note at the same time that these data on emotional status may be providing information in regard to the patients at particular risk for subsequent emotional problems in association with their illness. Thus, they may help to designate which men might be particular targets for special professional attention and support.

Third, patients should know how and to whom they can turn for help: to social workers, counselors, ministers, their friends or relatives, or to self-help groups. What is ironic and somewhat surprising is that the patients in our study made so little use of the wealth of social service agencies in their communities. Many patients may not know that these sources of aid and support are available to them. Thus, we may need to educate patients as well as physicians and to improve appropriate referrals to these agencies.

One salutory development in recent years is vigorous growth of the self-help movement. Self-help groups can provide most useful information and mutual support to one another and, with regard to many of the problems which patients experience, can be even more helpful than health professionals. Self-help groups can instruct their members in ways of getting additional needed services and in ways of negotiating the bureaucratic maze of the health care system. Professionals, for their part, have much to learn about the scope and services self-help groups may provide and how they can be enlisted in behalf of patients. In recent years, health professionals, increasingly, have referred their patients to self-help groups.

We know that friends and families are very important sources of help for many of the patients but that some patients are well integrated socially and others are not. Those who are relatively isolated at the beginning of their illness, in all likelihood, will possess few social resources a decade later. Physicians and medical social workers should work with patients to identify friends and relatives who may provide support, and, where necessary, should help patients establish early contact with other types of resources in the community.

Fourth, we must study why semiskilled and unskilled workers experience such high rates of mortality as heart patients. As the reasons for these rates are not clear, we can recommend that physicians watch these patients closely and pay particular attention to the specific requirements of their jobs and to the problems they experience in adhering to medical regimens.

Fifth, we may be reasonably confident that while executives and professionals have relatively favorable rates of survival, they are more likely to experience problems in connection with their work. They are more likely to feel that they are handicapped in their chances for promotion or advancement. In addition, men in the upper occupational categories are more likely to experience greater work stress and to cite emotional tension at work as a cause of their heart attack. Some realistic counseling may prove useful.

Even more, it may be necessary to encourage employers not to discriminate against the average heart patient. Our study does lend support to a policy of nondiscrimination: while the heart patient is coping with ongoing chronic disease, he is able to perform well and to fulfill his responsibilities. An unfair employment policy, indeed, may be the most serious problem some heart patients may encounter.

Sixth, the physician, or some other member of the health care team, should work with the patient's family, as well. Family members can be helpful in supporting the patient's effort to follow his medical regimen. Moreover, the patient's illness impacts on the family which, in turn, provides the emotional climate for the patient. Thus, the perspectives and approaches of family-oriented medicine are most appropriate for the heart patient.

If we are serious in meeting the varied needs of heart patients, we must ask how this concern is to be encompassed in the design of our health system of the future. In recent years, health planners have shown more appreciation of the larger social and psychological context of chronic illness. One manifestation of this was the decision a few years ago by the National Heart, Lung, and Blood Institute in establishing a Task Force on Rehabilitation of Coronary Patients, with a mandate to study the problem in *all* its aspects. How we design our national health insurance system will provide a true test of our commitment to the care of long-term chronic conditions. Do we place an important premium on health education, on social supports, and on the psychological and social needs of patients? What incentives will we provide to assure that the full range of patient needs are met?

How these questions and issues involving heart patients are handled are matters of much concern for all of us. From the personal point of view they are relevant, as most of the population will at some time develop heart disease or some other chronic disease condition, and each of us will be directly affected by the character of the resources and supports in the society. But beyond this, the care and support system for the chronically ill—and for other impaired and disadvantaged persons—is a measure of the morality and concern of the society as a whole, and these matters are therefore a responsibility of all of us.

NOTE

1. It should be pointed out, too, that the question was asked before the present rate of accelerated inflation.

APPENDIX A

I. THE BASE-LINE STUDY: WEEK 3, WEEK 7, AND YEAR 1

The selection of the initial study population for this longitudinal research was based on a series of medical and demographic criteria. The study population consisted of 345 men, who were previously well, who had suffered a first myocardial infarction, who were between the ages of 30 and 60, and who were discharged from the hospital after a "noncomplicated" hospitalization. The base-line study was initially located at the Harvard School of Public Health, and the research itself was carried out in the communities of Greater Boston and Worcester, Massachusetts. The study population consisted of men drawn from all socioeconomic levels. All were Caucasian. (A report of demographic characteristics appears later in this Appendix.)

A main principle in selection of the study population was that the patients should be previously well, i.e., that this first myocardial infarction should be their first significant illness. This was done inasmuch as we wished to rule out the possible effects of previous adjustment to major illness in our study of processes of recovery and rehabilitation following a heart attack.

To facilitate selection of the study population, a series of specific criteria were developed in order to arrive at a relatively homogeneous population from the medical standpoint: patients whose condition was generally similar in terms of severity and degree of complications. (For a detailed statement of selection criteria, see listing at end of this Appendix.)

When the study was originally designed, consultants and hospital officials indicated there would be no major difficulty finding cases that fit our strict criteria. Our experience revealed, however, that it is relatively rare to find mycardial infarction without previous significant illness in men in the age group specified. It eventually became necessary to obtain the cooperation of 26 hospitals in the areas of Greater Boston and Worcester, Massachusetts, in order to ensure a study population of sufficient size without unduly prolonging the case intake period.[1]

Medical Screening Procedures.

In order to maintain an effective and medically sound means of screening cases, special organizational arrangements were set up. These procedures were overseen and coordinated by the Medical Director of the project. In each of the participating hospitals a "contact physician" was appointed who was directly responsible to the Medical Director. The contact physician was usually a resident or a Fellow, although in several hospitals it was necessary to employ a private practitioner from the hospital staff.

The contact physician screened all new cardiac cases admitted to the hospital. If a patient fit criteria for the study, the contact physician completed a form which summarized essential details of the case, including the nature and severity of the patient's condition. The contact person also obtained permission from the patient's physician before asking the patient to participate in the study. The form was then reviewed by the Medical Director, and he made the final decision on acceptance of the case.

The contact physicians served in other ways as liaisons between the project and the hospital: their familiarity with the system minimized disruption of ward routine, and they had no difficulty gaining access to medical records. Further, they were able to answer whatever questions might arise on the part of patients, private practitioners, or project interviewers.

Cooperation from practicing physicians affiliated with the participating hospitals was excellent. At least 98% of the doctors approached by the contact physicians permitted their patients to be asked to participate in the study. While this method of finding and screening cases proved effective for our purposes, it was expensive in terms of money, administrative requirements, and paperwork.

Data Collection

Data were collected at each phase by means of a series of instruments. These were: (1) interview schedules administered to the patient and his wife or a close relative; (2) questionnaires completed by physicians; and (3) supplementary materials obtained through intensive case interview methods.

The heart patients were interviewed in a three-stage program during the base-line study. The first interview took place in the hospital about 18 days after admission and shortly before discharge. The second interview was conducted a month after the patient's discharge from the hospital. It was timed to intercept the patient while he was still in the early transitional period of coping with his new role as cardiac patient. The third interview was completed at 1 year after the date of initial hospital admission. This timing enabled examination of the level of performance of patients after a standardized period of adjustment to the illness.

Interviews were of the survey research type, consisting primarily of fixed alternative questions with a number of supplementary open-ended items. Interviews were conducted by social workers, each of whom held a Master of Social Work degree.

The first interview was designed to develop information concerning the patient's perception of his illness, his appraisal of potential problems of adjustment and future situation after discharge, and his plans for changes in work, family life, and activity patterns after his return home. The second and third interviews were designed to obtain information in regard to a series of major life areas, in addition to social identification and background data. Examples are: (1) work history and the impact of the heart attack on return to work, relationships at work, and on employment prospects and plans; (2) family relationships and the influence of the heart attack upon these; (3) medical care costs and their impact on family financial resources; (4) doctor-patient communication on the therapeutic regimen and level of compliance by the patient; (5) past, present, and prospective use of physician services, hospitals, and agencies for support and care; and (6) formal and informal memberships and associations. Other areas were: (7) reported symptoms of illness and of disability over time, and the incidence of rehospitalizations; (8) psychological characteristics of patients and their stability and change over time; (9) measures of subjective social stress; and (10) changes in religious views and in quality of life over time.

At the times of the Week 7 and Year 1 interviews with the patient, his wife was interviewed separately. If the patient was unmarried, widowed, or divorced, the interviews were held with a close relative living in the home. The spouse/relative interviews in many respects followed the same format as those instruments used with the patients. They were designed to elicit information on the patient's situation which he might be either unable or unwilling to furnish, and they provided another perspective on his life and problems from the viewpoint of an involved observer.

In addition to the interviews, data concerning the patients were also obtained from the physicians who provided their care. Physicians were asked to complete questionnaires at Week 7 and Year 1. The questionnaire items requested ratings of the health level and functional capacity of the patients, and assessments of their prognosis for the succeeding year. The questionnaires also contained items on the nature of instructions given to the patient in regard to such matters as physical activity, work, retirement, recreation, diet, drug therapy, and life style. Physicians were asked to make assessments of compliance by the patient.

Cooperation from physicians was excellent. Approximately 90% completed the questionnaires at each stage.

CASE DISTRIBUTIONS: AN ACCOUNTING FOR THE BASE-LINE STUDY

Case intake extended from July 1, 1965 through May 31, 1967, a period of 23 months. Since the interview program was designed to continue for a year beyond the last Week 3 interview, the entire period of data gathering, through the last interview, was approximately 3 years (July 1, 1965 through May 31, 1968).

Table A–1 presents the pattern of case losses for the entire base-line study period.

The Case Population at Week 3

A total of 556 men were referred from the 26 participating hospitals by the contact physicians. Although the criteria had been specified, the contact physicians tended to err on the side of referring all patients who might possibly be acceptable. Accordingly, thorough screening was carried out by the Medical Director for the project. The large majority of case rejections occurred on medical grounds. The final group of patients who completed first interviews numbered 414.

The Core Study Population: From Week 3 to Week 7

Data from the first interviews revealed that 32 of the 414 men had ailments not previously reported. Another 3 men became "geographically ineligible," having moved to locations outside the study area. These 35 men were eliminated from the study, reducing the population size to 379. During the period between the first and second interviews, 3 patients died and 18 men refused, directly or indirectly, to continue participating. These losses further reduced the population to 358 patients, all of whom completed the second interview. (See Table A–2 for categories of case losses.)

"Indirect refusal" is a term characterizing those patients who through various means avoided being reinterviewed. Their evasiveness finally led us to drop them from the study group. In Table A–1 this category also includes losses through staff decisions. The decision was made to excuse patients from participation in the few instances where further inquiry might lead to personal embarrassment or problems in family relationships.

Of the 358 men 13 were later found to be medically ineligible or inappropriate for inclusion, and they were accordingly omitted from the study population. This group included five men who were nonwhite. The criteria for the study population initially

Table A-1. Case Loss Progression in Base-line Study.

A. *COMPOSITION OF INITIAL STUDY POPULATION: WEEK 3*

Eligible:	Week 3 interviews completed,	74.6	(414)
	Transferred to Case Study*	1.8	(10)
	Refusals, outright and indirect	5.8	(32)
Ineligible:	Medically	15.3	(85)
	Geographically	2.5	(15)
		100%	(556)

*See *The Heart Patient Recovers* (1977), pages 44 and 391.

B. *PARTICIPATION AND CASE LOSS PATTERN AT WEEK 7*

Eligible:	Week 7 interviews completed:		
	"core" study group	83.3	(345)
	Refusals, outright and indirect	4.4	(18)
Deceased	between Week 3 and Week 7 interviews	1.2	(3)
Ineligible:	Medically	9.2	(40)
	Geographically	.7	(3)
	Nonwhites†	1.2	(5)
		100%	(414)

†Because the number of eligible nonwhites was small, the decision was made, for statistical reasons, to exclude them from the "core" study population.

C. *PARTICIPATION AND CASE LOSS PATTERN*
OF "CORE" STUDY GROUP AT YEAR 1

Eligible:	Year 1 interviews completed	84.9	(293)
	Refusals, outright and indirect	10.7	(37)
Deceased	between Week 7 and Year 1 interviews	3.8	(13)
Ineligible:	Medically	.3	(1)
	Geographically	.3	(1)
		100%	(345)

had included no stipulation concerning race, for it was hoped that sufficient numbers of whites and nonwhites would be obtained to permit meaningful analysis. Since so few nonwhites were found who fit the medical criteria, however, it was apparent that it would not be possible to make appropriate statistical comparisons and tests of significance. Hence, the decision was made to include only Caucasian men in the study.[2]

With these reductions, the final core population at Week 7 consisted of 345 men. This included those Caucasian men who completed Week 7 interviews and who fit criteria for health history, age, geographic location, and survival.

The Core Study Population: From Week 7 to Year 1

The study population at Year 1 included 293 of the 345 men in the core group. It contained approximately 88% of those who were living and eligible at the time. Of the 345 men 13 had died between the second and third interviews, 2 were deemed ineligible, and the other 37 men were lost through either outright or indirect refusals. Our experience suggests that some of these 37 patients refused because once they had recovered and became fully involved again with their lives, they were unwilling to be reminded in another interview of their earlier illness experience.

Case Attrition

In the cases of patients who died during the first year, information on the cause and circumstances of death was obtained by the Medical Director through questionnaires sent to their physicians.

In order to assess possible effects of case attrition in biasing our findings, a special analysis was carried out. Cases lost at Week 7 and Year 1 were compared with the rest of the study population in regard to such variables as age, marital status, religious affiliation, occupational and educational levels, social class, anticipated work status, and denial of the heart attack. No statistically significant differences were found between the participants and patients lost to the study through direct refusal, indirect refusal, or death. (For a definition of categories of cases lost to the project, see Table A–2.)

Spouse/Relative Interviews: Week 7 and Year 1

Of the Week 7 core population of 345 men, there were 325 cases in which a spouse or relative was potentially available for interview in the household. At Week 7, interviews were completed in 306 of these cases, including 289 with wives. Three potential respondents were physically or mentally ill, and the other 16 refused, directly or indirectly, to participate. Thus, there was 94% participation by spouse/relative respondents at Week 7.

Table A-2. Categories of Cases Lost to the Project

1. Ineligible:	*On medical grounds.* Does not fulfill medical criteria. Includes both mental and physical illness. Course of illness in the hospital was other than "noncomplicated."
	On geographic grounds. Comes from out of state or moves to distant location.
2. Deceased	
3. Refusal:	*Outright.* Overt rejection of continued participation by patient (or spouse/relative).
	Indirect. A residual category indicating possible oblique rejection of continued participation. For example, interview evaded, patient cannot be traced, opposition to patient's participation by wife directly or patient claims wife is reluctant to have him participate, evidence further inquiry might lead to personal embarrassment for the patient, etc.
4. Staff Decision on Eligibility:	So few nonwhites in the study after exclusions on basis of other criteria that, for statistical reasons, decision was made to exclude five eligible nonwhites.

At the time of the Year 1 interview, 240 of the 306 spouse/ relative respondents interviewed earlier participated again. Of the nonresponding 66, 42 were not contacted for an interview because there had been no Year 1 interview with the patient. (We interpreted refusals by patients as meaning that neither patient nor spouse/relative wanted to participate further, and we there-fore removed both from the study.) Three spouse/relative re-spondents no longer lived under the same roof with the patient, 4 were ill, and 17 refused participation, either indirectly or out-right. Some additional increments occurred, however. Six wives who had previously been unavailable for interview at Week 7 completed the Year 1 interview. Their number raised the spouse/ relative interview population to 246. This represents 92% parti-cipation by the spouse/relative respondents at Year 1.

Distributions in the "Core" Patient Population

As has been mentioned, the study population was selected on the basis of criteria suited for our particular research purposes: examining responses of men active in their careers to crisis of first serious illness. It was not designed to serve as a random sample of all heart patients. Rather, the emphasis was upon developing a relatively homogeneous population in terms of the criteria. Screening eliminated some of the effects of intervening variables, including those involving variation by previous illness pattern, sex, advanced age, and racial origins.

Although this population is not a "sample" in the scientific sense, the question of possible bias in selection was a source of continuing concern to the investigators. Hence, several types of efforts were made to ascertain whether the project was receiving notification of all cases fitting the criteria. First, the Medical Director repeatedly interviewed the contact physicians. All main-tained they were reporting every case that fit the criteria. Second, two of the Medical Directors served successively as contact physi-cians themselves for periods in certain participating hospitals. The number of cases they found was consistent with that re-ported by contact physicians in each of the hospitals given this special scrutiny.

Third, a special project was undertaken to explore possibili-ties of underreporting. A nurse was employed to review the records of all coronary cases admitted to three of the participating hospitals for the year immediately preceding the inception of the study. These institutions were: Massachusetts General Hospital, Newton-Wellesley Hospital, and the Boston Veterans' Administration Hospital. Data from this special study were analyzed by our medical consultant. His appraisal indicated that the number of cases obtained from these three hospitals during the study was approximately that which might have been predicted on the basis of actual admissions during the preceding year.

The case-finding procedures resulted in a study population of men who, in a general sense, appeared to fit the major characteristics of the geographic area in which they resided. Some indications of distributions in terms of selected demographic variables may be seen in Table A–3. It presents condensed tabulations reporting on the core population of 345 patients at Week 7.

II. THE LONG-TERM FOLLOW-UP STUDY: YEAR 8

A Year 8 interview extended the longitudinal approach and provided data on the heart patients approximately 7 years after Year 1 and 8 years after the first heart attack. Its purpose was to trace the initial study population and to obtain information on a broad series of areas in the long-term experience of coping with nearly a decade of chronic illness. The follow-up interview enabled comparison of the Year 8 data with the base-line materials, and the measurement of essentially the same phenomena in a systematic manner over time.

Data for the follow-up study were collected through two principal sources: (1) patient interviews, and (2) physician questionnaires.

Interviews with Patients

Patient interviews at Year 8 were similar in content and basic format to those carried out earlier at Week 7 and Year 1. They consisted of both fixed-alternative and open-ended questions. The same major areas of information were covered as in the earlier interviews, but appropriate adjustments in questions were

Table A-3. Distributions of Selected Demographic Variables in Core Population at Week 7. $N = 345$.

Age	Percent	N	Marital Status	Percent	N
30–39	9.8	34	Married	88.7	306
40–49	36.0	124	Never Married	5.2	18
50–59	54.1	187	Divorced, Widowed, Separated	6.1	21

Education	Percent	N	Hollingshead Index of Social Position Level	Percent	N
One Year of College or more	24.1	83	1, 2 (Highest)	15.7	54
			3	18.3	63
Four Years High School	32.2	111	4	44.0	152
			5	22.0	76
Three Years High School or Less	43.8	151			

Religion	Percent	N	Ethnic Origins*	Percent	N
Protestant	21.4	74	British-Old American	10.7	37
Catholic	59.7	206	Irish	19.7	68
Jewish	14.5	50	Italian	16.8	58
Other	4.3	15	Jewish	14.2	49
			Other and Mixed	38.6	133

*Patient was coded as being in a particular ethnic group if he responded that both parents were of that origin.

made to permit comparison with the base-line data. In addition, items were added in order to provide data on the period since Year 1 with special emphasis on the year immediately preceding the Year 8 interview. The new series of questions centered on changes in health care behavior, adjustment to aging, subjective perception of symptoms, and use of cash benefit programs and disability insurance. For example, to collect information concerning sources and amount of income, patients were presented with a checklist reviewing types of income, and amounts received during the past 12 months. Such items were included as wages or salary, rental income, Social Security disability benefits, Worker's Compensation, veterans benefits, private insurance disability benefits, etc.

The follow-up interview program began in 1974 and extended for approximately 1 year. In the initial interviewing program for the base-line study, case intake extended for a year and a half. Hence, between the first and last patients there was an interval of 18 months. When the year 8 interviews were carried out, it was necessary for reasons of financial expediency to condense the interviewing period, rather than wait a year and a half to see each man on the anniversary of his previous interview session in the base-line study.

Because of differences within the Year 8 population in regard to amount of time since Year 1, analyses were carried out to determine whether this factor had apparent significant effects on response patterns. The population was divided into three groups according to the length of the interval between the Year 1 and the Year 8 interviews, and comparisons were made to determine whether these groups differed significantly from each other on such variables as demographic traits, rehospitalizations, and smoking patterns. As no significant differences were found, the Year 8 population is treated here as a single group.

A few patients were either unwilling or unable to complete full Year 8 interviews. It was still possible to collect some basic information from these patients by means of a condensed form of the interview, which was completed either by mail or by telephone. Information gained from these "short forms" included current employment status, hospitalization experience, and receipt of Social Security benefits.

Because of limited funds, it was not possible to interview the wives at year 8.

Interviewers

For the follow-up study five interviewers were employed. All of these had attained at least a Master's degree in social work, had been specially trained for the project, and had worked on the earlier study. The field operation was located at Boston University. The Field Operations Supervisor was Roberta Idelson. She directed the activities of the interviewers, tracked down patients, kept records, and supervised quality control in the interviewing program.

Physician Questionnaires

In addition to the interviews, data concerning the patients were obtained from either the patient's private physician, or the physician serving as his main source of care. Through request of the Medical Director, each doctor was asked to complete a mail questionnaire at Year 8. These dealt with the doctor's assessment of the patient's current cardiac status, cardiac prognosis, and total health status, including level of impairment.

There were 186 patients for whom adequate information was available to send the questionnaire. Eighty-five percent of the doctors of these patients returned questionnaires. Eleven of these physicians returned questionnaires which were incomplete, because of lack of sufficient current information on the patient. In the cases of a small remaining group of patients, questionnaires were never sent. The main reason was that the patients indicated they had no physician. Table A–4 presents a summary of data on return of physician questionnaires at Year 8.

Data Processing

While the interviewing program was still in progress, coding instructions were developed for the interview and the physician questionnaire. This task was a substantial one; there were 660 variables available to code from both instruments. A staff of nine

Table A-4. Physician Questionnaire Return Rate Summary at Year 8*

Physician Questionnaire Return Rate: Category 1 (N = 175)

N	Percent	Disposition of Questionnaire
148	84.57	Returned completed
27	15.43	Never returned, even after follow-up
175	100.00	

Physician Questionnaire Return Rate: Category 2 (N = 30)

N	Percent	Disposition of Questionnaire
2	6.7	Returned incomplete; physician retired
7	23.3	Returned incomplete; physician does not consider himself able to answer. Physician has not seen patient recently.
2	6.7	Returned incomplete; physician does not consider himself able to answer on cardiac status. Physician is a neurologist or other specialist.
12	40.0	Never sent; patient has no physician
2	6.7	Never sent; unable to use patient information to locate physician
3	10.0	No response/uncodable
2	6.7	Never sent; patient refused to give permission
30	100.1†	

*Percentages do not sum to 100.0 due to rounding.

†The table represents the return rate of the Year 8 physician questionnaires. The pattern of response is tabulated according to two different categories of physician response: (1) Physician returned questionnaire or indicated a refusal through direct or indirect means (N=175); (2) physician did not complete questionnaire for a series of reasons other than personal direct or indirect refusal, such as lack of recent contact with patient, retirement of physician, statement by patient that he had no physician, and related reasons (N=30).

persons was employed part time to perform the coding. In order to ensure minimal error, a 100% check was done on all coding.

The product of data collection, a large body of coded information, was keypunched, verified, and stored on 15 decks of

IBM cards, or 15 80-column cards per patient. These cards were then written to tape for use on the Univac 1106 in the Data Services Division of the University of Connecticut Health Center. Analysis was carried out through use of SPSS (Statistical Package for the Social Sciences).

The Core Study Population: From Year 1 to Year 8

Most case losses between Year 1 and Year 8 were due to patient deaths ($N = 69$). There was only one man from the core Year 1 population for whom no information was available; this was because he had left the country. Two-hundred and five patients completed full Year 8 interviews. Basic data was obtained from 18 others by means of either the short form of the interview or other mail or phone contact. See Table A–5a for a summary of cases lost, based on the core population at Year 1.

The Core Study Population: From Week 7 to Year 8

At Year 8 we also attempted to collect information on men who had been included in the core population at Week 7, but not at Year 1 ($N = 52$). Twenty-three men from this group were deceased at Year 8. Another 20 patients refused to be interviewed, but 9 men provided some data either through the condensed form of the interview or other contact. Table A–5b summarizes case loss from Week 7 to Year 8.

Distributions in the "Core" Patient Population at Year 8

Distributions on selected demographic variables were computed for the core population of 205 patients at Year 8 (See Table A–6). This was done in order to determine if the major characteristics of the study population had changed substantially due to case losses since the original selection of the base-line population. Table A–6 can be compared with Table A–3, which presents the distributions of the same demographic variables in the core population at Week 7.

The comparison reveals that relatively little change had occurred in the study population in terms of the percentage distributions shown. The one exception is, of course, the age variable.

**Table A-5a. Participation and Case Loss Pattern at Year 8
Interview Based Upon "Core" Population at Year 1
(N = 293).**

	Percent	Percent of Surviving Patients at Year 8	N
Eligible: Year 8 interviews completed	70.0	91.5	205
Short forms completed*	3.4	4.5	10
Phone/letter contact†	2.7	3.5	8
Not traceable‡	.4	.5	1
Deceased between Year 1 and Year 8 interviews	23.5	—	69
	100.0	100.0	293

**Table A-5b. Participation and Case Loss Pattern at Year 8
Interview Based Upon "Core" Population at Week 7
(N = 345).**

	Percent	N
Eligible: Year 8 interviews completed	59.4	205
Short forms completed*	5.2	18
Phone/letter contact†	2.6	9
Refusals, outright and indirect§	6.1	21
Deceased: from Year 1 population	20.0	69
from Week 7 population	6.7	23
	100.0	345

*A few patients were either unwilling or unable to complete full Year 8 interviews, but completed a condensed form.
†A small number of patients were resistant to participation in either the complete or condensed form of the Year 8 interview, but were able to provide some information about themselves by letter or telephone.
‡A single patient was not traceable. He had left the United States some years previously.
§For definition of category, see Table A-2.

Table A-6. Distributions of Selected Demographic Variables in Core Population at Year 8. N = 205.

Age	Percent	N	Marital Status	Percent	N
40–44	4.9	10	Married	87.8	180
45–49	8.3	17	Never Married	4.9	10
50–54	19.5	40	Divorced,	7.3	15
55–59	24.4	50	Widowed, Sepa-		
60–64	25.4	52	rated		
65–70	17.5	36			

Education	Percent	N	Hollingshead Index of Social Position Level	Percent	N
One Year of College or more	28.8	59	1, 2 (Highest)	17.6	36
			3	20.5	42
Four Years High School	30.2	62	4	44.4	91
Three Years High School or Less	41.0	84	5	17.6	36

Religion	Percent	N	Ethnic Origins*	Percent	N
Protestant	23.4	48	British-Old American	11.2	23
Catholic	56.6	116	Irish	20.5	42
Jewish	16.1	33	Italian	14.2	29
Other	3.9	8	Jewish	15.6	32
			Other and Mixed	38.5	79

*See footnote in Table A-3.

Notes

1. Participating hospitals were: Beth Israel, Boston City, Boston Veterans Administration, Brockton, Cambridge City, Carney, Faulkner, Framingham-Union, Lynn, Malden, Massachusetts General, Mt. Auburn, New England Baptist, New England Deaconess, New England Medical Center, Newton-Wellesley, Peter Bent Brigham, Quincy City, St. Elizabeth's, St. Vincent's (Worcester), United States Public Health Service, University, Waltham, West Roxbury Veterans Administration, Worcester City, and Worcester Memorial.

2. See also *The Heart Patient Recovers* (1977), pp. 383–384.

Listing of Selection Criteria

Criteria for screening patients who had symptoms indicative of, or disease predisposing to, myocardial infarction were developed by the medical directors for the project. They are as follows:

Arteriosclerotic Heart Disease

Those with suspected but unconfirmed angina pectoris of any duration will be accepted into the study.

Patients with definite angina pectoris of 1 month's duration or less will be accepted into the study.

Patients with definite diagnosed angina pectoris of greater than 1 month's duration will be excluded from the study.

Patients with suspected but unconfirmed coronary insufficiency, congestive heart failure, or previous myocardial infarction will be excluded.

Other Heart Disease

No patient with heart disease other than arteriosclerotic disease diagnosed previously to myocardial infarction will be included in the study.

No patient with heart disease other than arteriosclerotic disease which is diagnosed at the time of the infarction will be included.

Diseases Predisposing to Arteriosclerotic Heart Disease

Diabetes: Patients with diabetes diagnosed at the time of the myocardial infarction will be accepted into the study.

Patients who had diagnosed diabetes at the time of the myocardial infarction and are being treated by diet, oral hypoglycemics, and insulin will be excluded from the study.

Hypertension: Patients with hypertension first diagnosed at the time of the myocardial infarction will be included in the study.

Patients who have had diagnosed hypertension but have not received treatment for the disease will be included in the study.

All those patients who had had previously diagnosed hypertension which required therapy will be excluded from the study.

Gout: Patients will be accepted if the diagnosis of gout was made at the time of the infarction but not if made previously.

Hypercholesterolemia, Hyperlipedemia: Patients will be accepted with these disorders if the diagnosis had previously not been confirmed or suspected at the time of the infarction.

Hyperthyroidism: Patients will be accepted into the study if the diagnosis of primary hyperthyroidism is made at the time of the infarction.

Patients with secondary hyperthyroidism will be excluded from the study.

Acceptance of Patients With "Noncomplicated" Clinical Course: Only those patients whose clinical course during first hospitalization was "without complications" will be accepted for the interview program.

Noncardiovascular Disease: Patients who had had a well-defined, discrete episode of noncardiac disease that did not require continuing medical attention were eligible for the study if the episode had occurred more than 3 years prior to the first myocardial infarction.

APPENDIX B

MULTIPLE REGRESSION ANALYSIS OF HEALTH OUTCOMES AND DEMOGRAPHIC SOCIAL AND PSYCHOLOGICAL "PREDICTOR" VARIABLES

Multiple regression analysis is a general statistical technique which allows for the examination of the common variances between a set of independent or predictor variables and a criterion variable (dependent variable). In this case, our interest was in two types of dependent variables: (1) mortality during the period from Year 1 to Year 8; and (2) mortality and/or morbidity measures during the Year 1 to Year 8 period. A list of the dependent variables (criterion variables) and the independent variables (predictor variables) appears at the end of this Appendix.

The multiple regression analysis addressed three principal questions in connection with the data from the study population:

1. Given a total set of variables, what sort of prediction with a criterion variable is possible?
2. If prediction is possible, which combinations of sets of variables improve prediction?

3. What is the contribution of individual predictor variables to (a) the respective subsets of predictor variables, and (b) the total pool of predictor variables?

First, we address the issue of mortality and its possible "predictors," making use of social, demographic, and illness-type antecedent variables. The results from the analysis neither confirm nor refute previous nonparametric analyses with these data. Though multiple correlations were low, this could be a reflection of failure to meet the underlying assumptions of the multiple regression model, or it could be due to a true lack of interrelationships.

With regard to mortality/morbidity criterion variables and their possible antecedents, the findings are perhaps more illuminating. The "illness level" variables, measured as of Year 1, appear to make the most substantial contribution to the prediction of Year 8 mortality/morbidity outcomes. The social and demographic variables were not of key importance. As noted in Chapter 2, these findings are consistent with those derived from nonparametric analysis. In sum, these results from multiple regression analysis do not make contributions beyond those already available through nonparametric methods.

I. *Independent Variables Grouped by Type of Variable*
    Demographic

Age	Six levels: 30–34, 35–39, 40–44, 45–49, 50–54, 55–60.
Educational Level	Seven levels: Graduate professional training, college graduate, partial college, high school graduate, partial high school, junior high school, grade school
Pre-illness Occupational Level	Six levels: Executives and professionals, managers, administrative personnel, clerical and sales workers, skilled workers, semi-skilled and unskilled workers.

Illness Level

Rehospitalization Between Initial Release and Year 1	Two levels: Rehospitalized for coronary heart disease, not rehospitalized for coronary heart disease.
Year 1 Physician Rating of Functional Health Status	Three levels: No significant impairment, moderate impairment, severe impairment.
Year 1 Total Number of Symptoms	Eight levels: None, one, two, three, four, five, six, seven or more.
Year 1 Level of Severity of Illness	Three levels: Not rehospitalized, no illness; not rehospitalized but rated ill by physician; rehospitalized for heart disease or other condition.
Year 1 Depressive Reaction	Two levels: yes, no.
Rehospitalization between Year 1 and Year 8	Two levels: Rehospitalized for coronary heart disease, not rehospitalized for coronary heart disease.
Year 8 Physician Cardiac Prognosis	Four levels: Good, good with therapy, fair with therapy, guarded despite therapy.

Pre-illness Psychological Self-Ratings (As Rated at Week 7)

22 Items (see Chapter 7)	Five levels: Not at all, a little, somewhat, considerably, very much.

II. *Dependent Variables at Year 8*
     Mortality
     1)   Deceased (Year 1 to Year 8)
     2)   Survivors (Alive at Year 8)

Mortality/Morbidity
1) Deceased (Year 1 to Year 8)
2) Survived with hospitalization for coronary heart disease between Year 1 and Year 8
3) Survived without rehospitalization for coronary heart disease between Year 1 and Year 8

Number of Activities Which Patient Has Trouble Performing
Range: 0 to 4

Number of Flights of Stairs Patient Can Climb Without Discomfort
Range: 0 to 6 or more

Number of Symptoms Which Patient Experienced During Preceding Month
Range: 0 to 14

Number of Days in Preceding Month On Which Patient Experienced Pain or Discomfort
Range: 0 to 25 or more

APPENDIX C

I. Master List of Independent Variables Used in Nonparametric Analysis of Morbidity/Mortality at Year 8
    1) Age of patient at Week 7
    2) Pre-illness occupation of patient
    3) Educational level of patient
    4) Ethnic origin of patient
    5) Year 1 rehospitalization history:
        a) Rehospitalized for heart condition
        b) Rehospitalized for other condition
        c) Not rehospitalized
    6) Illness severity at Year 1:
        a) Rehospitalized
        b) Not rehospitalized, but has developed disorders associated with arteriosclerotic heart disease, as assessed by physician.
        c) Not rehospitalized, and has not developed disorders associated with arteriosclerotic heart disease
    7) Physician rating of functional health status at Year 1:
        a) No significant impairment

   b) Moderate impairment
   c) Severe impairment
  8) Reported symptoms by patient at Year 1:
   a) None
   b) One
   c) Two
   d) Three
   e) Four
   f) Five
   g) Six
   h) Seven or more
  9) Patient's report of depression or discouragement over illness at Year 1:
   a) Yes
   b) No
  10) to 21) Psychological characteristics as reported by patient (for pre-illness period)[1]
   a) Not at all
   b) Medium
   c) High

II. Master List of All Dependent Variables Measuring Disability

1. Number of activities patient has difficulty performing (one to four)
2. Number of flights of stairs patient can climb without difficulty (none to six or more)
3. Number of days in past month patient unable to do usual work at home or on the job because of pain or discomfort (none to 16 or more)
4. Number of days in past month patient unable to do usual work at home or on the job because of pain or discomfort due to heart condition (none to 16 or more)
5. Number of days in past month patient spent ill in bed (none to 26 or more)
6. Number of days patient spent ill in bed due to his heart condition in past year (none to 26 or more)
7. Number of days patient spent ill in bed due to nonheart causes in past year (none to 26 or more)

III. Master List of All Dependent Variables Measuring Illness Symptoms
   1. to 17. Patient's self report of the frequency of pain or discomfort during the past month (not at all to three times or more)
      1. Getting tired easily
      2. Chest pain
      3. Breathlessness
      4. Feeling heart is pounding or skipping a beat
      5. Swelling of the feet or ankles
      6. Sleeplessness
      7. Restlessness or nervousness
      8. Upset stomach
      9. Headaches
      10. General aches or pains
      11. Loss of appetite
      12. Hands or feet shaking
      13. Spells of dizziness
      14. Fainting spells
      15. Cold sweats
      16. Pains from arthritis
      17. Crying spells
      18. Number of symptoms (items 1 to 17) mentioned once, twice, or three times (none to 15 or more)
      19. Number of days in past month patient experienced pain or discomfort from symptoms (none to 25 or more)
      20. Number of emergency room, clinic, or outpatient visits (none to 21 or more)

NOTE

1. Items were: sense of duty, gets angry easily, feelings easily hurt, nervous or irritable, moody, likes responsibility, easily excited, easily depressed, being in a hurry, being ambitious, being hard driving, and puts in a lot of effort.

APPENDIX D

ANTECEDENT, PRIMARY, AND SECONDARY INDEX VARIABLE VALUES.

I. *Antecedent and Social Identity Variables*

    a.   Age at Year 1

        1 = Old (50–60);
        2 = Middle (40–49);
        3 = Young (30–39)

    b.   Pre-Illness and Year 8 Occupation (Excludes currently retired men)

        1 = Executives and Professionals;
        2 = Administrative and Clerical Personnel, White-Collar;
        3 = Skilled Laborers;
        4 = Semiskilled or Unskilled Laborers

        Pre-Illness Occupation (2 levels)

        1 = Professional, White-collar, or Skilled Blue-Collar;
        2 = Semiskilled or Unskilled Blue-Collar

c. Education

1 = 1 Year of College or More;
2 = High School Graduate;
3 = Less than High School

d. Year 8 Total Family Income

1 = $20,000 or Above;
2 = $15,000–$19,999;
3 = $12,500–$14,999;
4 = $10,000–$12,499;
5 = $7,500–9,999; 6 = $7,499 or Less

e. Year 8 Marital Status

1 = Married; 2 = Not Married

f. Year 1, Year 8 Marital Happiness

1 = Very Happy; 2 = Happy;
3 = Less Than Happy

g. Year 8 Index of Marital Disagreement

1 = High (3 or More);
2 = Medium (1–2);
3 = Low (None)

h. Year 8 Index of Job Dissatisfaction, Very Dissatisfied or Dissatisfied

1 = 4 or more; 2 = 1–3;
3 = None

i. Year 1, Year 8 Index of Work Stress

1 = High (3–4); 2 = Low (1–2);
3 = None

j. Year 8 Frequency of Lifting Heavy Weights at Work

1 = Frequently; 2 = Sometimes;
3 = Rarely or Never

k. Year 1, Year 8 Index of Social Participation

1 = High (Once a Week or More);
2 = Low (Less Than Once A Week)

l. Year 8 Membership in Clubs

1 = 3 or More; 2 = Two;
3 = One; 4 = None

m. Year 8 Frequency of Church Attendance

1 = More Than Once A Month;
2 = 1 Month or Less;
3 = Never

n. Year 8 Importance of Religion

1 = Important; 2 = Not Important

o. Year 1, Year 8 Frequen-   1 = Frequently; 2 = Sometimes;
cy of Walks   3 = Rarely or Never

p. Presence of a Confidant   1 = Yes, 2 = No
at Week 7, Year 8

q. Week 7, Year 1 Gains   1 = Yes, 2 = No
from the Illness

r. Week 7, Year 1 Life   1 = Beyond Ambitions; 2 = Close
Goal Achievement   to Ambitions;
  3 = Behind Ambitions

s. Year 1 Depressive Reac-   1 = Yes; 2 = No
tion

t. Year 1 Physician Rating   1 = No Significant Impairment;
of Functional Health   2 = Moderate Impairment;
Status   3 = Severe Impairment

u. Week 7, Year 1 Subjective Stress Items
(A) Nervous strain in daily activities
(B) Generally tense and nervous
1 = Fairly or Very Well; 2 = Not Very Well or Not At All

v. Pre-Illness Psychological Factor Scores (in Terciles):
(A) Emotional Lability   1 = High; 2 = Medium; 3 = Low
(B) Ambition
(C) Dominance

w. Religious Affiliation:
(A) Protestant   1 = Protestant; 2 = Other
(B) Catholic   1 = Catholic; 2 = Other
(C) Jewish   1 = Jewish; 2 = Other

II. Primary Index Variables

a.   Physician Rating   1 = No Significant
    of Functional   Impairment; 2 = Moderate
    Health Status   Impairment; 3 = Severe
      Impairment

b. Satisfaction With Life Situation — 1 = Very Satisfied; 2 = Satisfied; 3 = Not Satisfied

c. 1) Work- Retirement Status A — 1 = "Normal" Career: Employed or retired; 2 = "Illness-Affected" Career: Unemployed or retired

2) Current Work Status B (Men Eligible for Work Force) — 1 = Employed; 2 = Unemployed

III. Secondary Index Variables

a. Index of Symptoms — 1 = High (5 or More); 2 = Low (0–4)

b. Subjective Stress Scale — 1 = High; 2 = Moderate; 3 = Low

c. Depressive Reaction — 1 = Yes; 2 = No

d. Gains from the Illness — 1 = Yes; 2 = No

e. Positive Change in Attitude Toward Life — 1 = Positive; 2 = No Change; 3 = Other Than Positive Change

f. Achievement of Life Goals — 1 = Beyond Ambitions; 2 = Close to Ambitions; 3 = Behind Ambitions

REFERENCES

Aday, L. A., & Andersen, R. *Access to medical care,* Ann Arbor: University of Michigan Press, 1975.

Aday, L. A., & Eichhorn, R. C. *The utilization of health services: Indices and correlates—a research bibliography* (DHEW Publication No. (HSM) 73–3003). Washington, D.C.: U.S. Department of Health, Education, and Welfare, December, 1972.

Aguilera, D., & Messick, J. M. *Crisis intervention—theory and methodology,* St. Louis: C. V. Mosby Co., 1974.

Alexander, F. *Psychosomatic medicine,* New York: W. W. Norton and Company, 1950.

Andersen, R. *A behavioral model of families' use of health services* (Research Series No. 25, Center for Health Administration Studies). Chicago: University of Chicago Press, 1968.

Andersen, R., Lion, J., & Anderson, O. W. *Two decades of health services,* Cambridge, Mass.: Ballinger, 1976.

Andersen, R., et al., *Medical care use in Sweden and the United States—a comparative analysis of systems and behavior* (Research Series No. 27, Center for Health Administration Studies). Chicago: University of Chicago Press, 1970.

Anderson, O. W., & Andersen, R. Patterns of use of health services. In H.

Freeman et al. (Eds.), *Handbook of medical sociology*. Englewood Cliffs, N.J.: Prentice-Hall, 1972, pp. 386–406.

Antonovsky, A. Social class, life expectancy and overall mortality. *Milbank Memorial Fund Quarterly*, 1967, *45*, 31–73.

Atchley, R. C. *The social forces in later life: An introduction to social gerontology*. Belmont, Calif.: Wadsworth Publishing Company, 1972.

Basch, M. F. Toward a theory that encompasses depression: A revision of existing causal hypotheses in psychoanalysis. In E. J. Anthony & T. Benedek (Eds.), *Depression and human existence*. Boston: Little, Brown and Company, 1975, pp. 485–534.

Becker, J. *Depression: Theory and research*. Washington, D.C.: V. H. Winston and Sons, 1974.

Becker, M. H. Psychosocial aspects of health-related behavior. In H. Freeman, S. Levine, & L. Reeder (Eds.), *Handbook of medical sociology*. Englewood Cliffs, N.J.: Prentice-Hall, 1979.

Becker, M. H., et al. Predicting mothers' compliance with pediatric medical regimens. *Journal of Pediatrics*, 1972, *81*, 843–854.

Becker, M. H., et al. A new approach to explaining sick-role behavior in low-income populations. *American Journal of Public Health*, 1974, *64*, 205–216.

Becker, M. H., & Maiman, L. A. Sociobehavioral determinants of compliance with health and medical care recommendations. *Medical Care*, 1975, *13*, 10–24.

Becker, M. H., et al. Selected psychosocial models and correlates of individual health-related behaviors. *Medical Care*, 1977, *15*, 27–46.

Bengtsson, C., Hallstrom, T., & Tibblin, G. Social factors, stress experience, and personality traits in women with ischemic heart disease, compared to the population sample of women. *Acta Medica Scandinavica* (Supplementum), 1973, *549*, 82–92.

Bibring, G. L. The mechanism of depression. In P. Greenacre (Ed.), *Affective disorders*. New York: International Universities Press, 1953, pp. 13–48.

Bice, T. W., & White, K. L. Cross-national comparative research on the utilization of medical services. *Medical Care*, 1971, *9*, 253–271.

Binstock, R. H., & Shanas, E. (Eds.). *Handbook of aging and the social sciences*. New York: Van Nostrand Reinhold Company, 1976.

Blackwell, B. Patient compliance, *New England Journal of Medicine*, 1973, *289*, 249–253.

Blau, Z. S. *Old age in a changing society*. New York: New Viewpoints, 1973.

Booth, P. *Social security in America*. Ann Arbor, Mich.: Institute of Labor and Industrial Relations, 1973.

Bruhn, J. G. et al. A psycho-social study of surviving male coronary patients and controls followed over nine years. *Journal of Psychosomatic Research*, 1971, *15*, 305–313.

Buell, J. C., & Eliot, R. S. Stress and cardiovascular disease. *Modern Concepts of Cardiovascular Disease*, 1979, *48*, 19–24.

Burgess, E. W., & Wallin, P. *Engagement and marriage*. Chicago: J. B. Lippincott, 1953.

Butler, R. *Why survive? Being old in America*. New York: Harper and Row, 1975.

Butler, R., & Lewis, M. *Aging and mental health: Positive psychosocial approaches*. St. Louis: C. V. Mosby Company, 1977.

Carp, F. M. (Ed.). *Retirement*. New York: Behavioral Publications, Inc., 1972.

Cath, S. H. The orchestration of disengagement. *International Journal of Aging and Human Development*, 1975, *6*, 199–213.

Comstock, G. W. Fatal arteriosclerotic heart disease, water hardness at home, and socioeconomic characteristics. *American Journal of Epidemiology*, 1971, *94*, 1–10.

Croog, S. H. The family as a source of stress. In S. Levine & N. A. Scotch (Eds.), *Social stress*. Chicago: Aldine Press, 1970, pp. 20–57.

Croog, S. H. Problems of barriers in the rehabilitation of heart patients: Social and psychological aspects. *Cardiac Rehabilitation*, 1975, *6*, 27–30.

Croog, S. H. Social aspects of rehabilitation after myocardial infarction: A selective review. In N. K. Wenger & H. K. Hellerstein (Eds.), *Rehabilitation of the coronary patient*. New York: Wiley and Sons, 1978, pp. 255–268.

Croog, S. H., & Fitzgerald, E. F. Subjective stress and serious illness of a spouse: Wives of heart patients. *Journal of Health and Social Behavior*, 1978, *19*, 166–178.

Croog, S. H., Koslowsky, M., & Levine, S. Personality self-perceptions of male heart patients and their wives: Issues of congruence and "coronary personality." *Perceptual and Motor Skills*, 1976, *43*, 927–937.

Croog, S. H., & La Voie, L. Depressive reaction and heart disease: An eight year longitudinal study. 1980, mimeo.

Croog, S. H., & Levine, S. Religion, secularism and personal crisis: A report on heart patients. *Social Science and Medicine*, 1972, *6*, 17–36.

Croog, S. H., & Levine, S. *The heart patient recovers.* New York: Human Sciences Press, 1977.

Croog, S. H., Lipson, A., & Levine, S. Help patterns in severe illness: The role of kin network and non-family resources. *Journal of Marriage and the Family*, 1972, *34*, 32–41.

Croog, S. H., & Richards, N. P. Health beliefs and smoking patterns in heart patients and their wives: A longitudinal study. *American Journal of Public Health*, 1977, *67*, 921–930.

Croog, S. H., Shapiro, D. S., & Levine, S. Denial among male heart patient. *Psychosomatic Medicine*, 1971, *33*, 385–397.

Cumming, E., & Henry, W. E. *Growing old. The process of disengagement.* New York: Basic Books, 1961.

Cuskey, W. R., et al. Predicting attrition during the outpatient detoxification of narcotic addicts. *Medical Care*, 1971, *9*, 108–116.

Davis, M. S. Variations in patients' compliance with doctors' orders: Analysis of congruence between survey responses and results of empirical investigations. *Journal of Medical Education*, 1966, *41*, 1037–1048.

Davis, M. S. Physiologic, psychological and demographic factors in patient compliance with doctors' orders. *Medical Care*, 1968, *6*, 115–122.

Davis, M. S., & Eichhorn, R. L. Compliance with medical regimens: A panel study. *Journal of Health and Human Behavior*, 1963, *4*, 240–249.

Dawber, T. R., & Kannel, W. B. Current status of coronary prevention: Lessons from the Framingham Study. *Preventive Medicine*, 1972, *1*, 499–512.

Dembroski, T. M., Weiss, S. M., Shields, J. L., Haynes, S., & Feinleib, M. (Eds.). *Coronary-prone behavior.* New York: Springer-Verlag, 1978.

Doehrman, S. Psycho-social aspects of recovery for coronary heart disease: A review. *Social Science and Medicine*, 1977, *11*, 199–218.

Donabedian, A. Models for organizing the delivery of personal health services and criteria for evaluating them. *Milbank Memorial Fund Quarterly*, 1972, *50*, 103–154.

Dreyfuss, F., Dasberg, H., & Assael, M. I. The relationship of myocardial infarction to depressive illness. *Psychotherapy and Psychosomatics*, 1969, *17*, 73–81.

Dunbar, F. *Mind and body: Psychosomatic medicine.* New York: Random House, 1948.

Dunbar, J. M., & Stunkard, A. J. Adherence to diet and drug regimen. In R. Levy et al. (Eds.), *Nutrition, lipids and coronary heart disease.* New York: Raven Press, 1979.

Eastwood, M. R., & Trevelyan, H. Stress and coronary heart disease. *Journal of Psychosomatic Research.* 1971, *15*, 289–292.

Engel, G. L., & Ader, R. Psychological factors in organic disease. *Mental Health Program Reports,* 1967, *1*, 1–25.

Epstein, L. J. Depression in the elderly. *Journal of Gerontology,* 1976, 278–282.

Fann, W. E., Wheless, J. C. Depression in elderly patients. *Southern Medical Journal,* 1975, *68*, 468–472.

Fieve, R. R. (Ed.). *Depression in the 1970's: Modern theory and research.* Amsterdam: Excerpta Medica, 1971.

Finlayson, A., & McEwen, J. *Coronary heart disease and patterns of living.* New York: Prodist, 1977.

Friedman, M. The modification of type A behavior in post-infarction patients. *American Heart Journal,* 1979, *97*, 551–560.

Friedman, M., & Rosenman, R. H. *Type A behavior and your heart.* New York: Knopf, 1974.

Garrity, T. Vocational adjustments after the first myocardial infarction: Comparative assessment of several variables suggested in the literature. *Social Science and Medicine,* 1973, *7*, 705–717.

Gordis, L. Methodologic issues in the measurement of patient compliance. In D. L. Sackett & R. B. Haynes (Eds.), *Compliance with therapeutic regimens.* Baltimore, Md.: The Johns Hopkins University Press, 1976, pp. 51–66.

Gordon, J. B. A disengaged look at disengagement theory. *International Journal of Aging and Human Development,* 1975, *6*, 215–227.

Haber, L. D. The effect of age and disability on access to public income-maintenance programs. *Social security survey of the disabled: 1966.* Washington, D.C.: United States Department of Health, Education and Welfare, Social Security Administration, July, 1968.

Haber, L. D. Age and capacity devaluation. *Journal of Health and Social Behavior,* 1970, *11*, 167–182.

Hackett, T. P., & Cassem, N. H. Psychological adaptation to convalescence in myocardial infarction patients. In J. P. Naughton & H. K.

Hellerstein (Eds.), *Exercise testing and exercise training in coronary heart disease.* New York: Academic Press, 1973, pp. 253–262.

Hammermeister, K., DeRowen, T., English, M., & Dodge, H. Effect of surgical versus medical therapy on return to work in patients with coronary artery disease. *American Journal of Cardiology,* 1979, *44,* 105–111.

Hammond, E. C., & Garfinkel, L. Smoking habits of men and women. *Journal of the National Cancer Institute,* 1961, *27,* 419–421, 426.

Hammond, E. C., & Garfinkel, L. The influence of health on smoking habits. *National Cancer Institute Monograph,* 1963, *19,* 269–285.

Haynes, S. G., & Feinleib, M. Women, work and coronary heart disease: Prospective findings from the Framingham Heart Study. *American Journal of Public Health,* 1980, *70,* 133–141.

Haynes, S. G., Feinleib, M., & Kannel, W. B. The relationship of psychosocial factors to coronary heart disease in the Framingham Study: III. Eight-year incidence of cornary heart disease. *American Journal of Epidemiology,* 1980, *111,* 37–58.

Haynes, S. G., Feinleib, M., Levine, S., Scotch, N., & Kannel, W. B. The relationship of psychosocial factors to coronary heart disease in the Framingham Study: II. Prevalence of coronary heart disease. *American Journal of Epidemiology,* 1978b, *107,* 384–401.

Haynes, S. G., Levine, S., Scotch, N., Feinleib, M., & Kannel, W. B. The relationship of psychosocial factors to coronary heart disease in the Framingham Study: I. Methods and risk factors. *American Journal of Epidemiology,* 1978a, *107,* 362–383.

Hochbaum, G. M. *Public participation in medical screening programs: A sociopsychological study* (Public Health Service Publication No. 572). Washington, D.C.: United States Government Printing Office, 1958.

Hollingshead, A. B. *Two factor index of social position.* New Haven, Conn.: privately printed, 1957.

House, J. S. Occupational stress as a precursor to coronary disease. In W. D. Gentry & R. B. Williams, Jr. (Eds.), *Psychological aspects of myocardial infarction and coronary care.* St. Louis: The C. V. Mosby Company, 1975, pp. 24–36.

Howards, I., & Brehm, H. P. The ecology of disability: Analysis of state population and SSDI program administration characteristics as they relate to state rates of disability. Report submitted by Department of Political Science, University of Massachusetts, Amherst, Massachusetts to Office of Research and Statistics, Social Security Administration, Baltimore, Maryland, February, 1977.

Hrubec, Z., & Zukel, W. J. Socioeconomic differentials in prognosis following episodes of coronary heart disease. *Journal of Chronic Diseases*, 1971, *23*, 881–889.

Jenkins, C. D. Psychologic and social precursors of coronary disease. *New England Journal of Medicine*, 1971, *284*, 244–255, 307–317.

Jenkins, C. D. Recent evidence supporting psychologic and social risk factors for coronary disease. *New England Journal of Medicine*, 1976, *294*, 987–994, 1033–1038.

Jenkins, C. D. Epidemiological studies of the psychosomatic aspects of coronary heart disease. *Advances in Psychosomatic Medicine*, 1977, *9*, 1–19.

Jenkins, C. D. Behavioral risk factors in coronary artery disease. *Annual Review of Medicine*, 1978a, *29*, 543–562.

Jenkins, C. D. Low education: A risk factor for death. *The New England Journal of Medicine*, 1978, *299*, 95–97.

Jenkins, C. D., Hurst, M. W., & Rose, R. M. Life changes: Do people really remember? *Archives of General Psychiatry*, 1979, *36*, 379–384.

Jenkins, C. D., Zyzanski, S. J. & Rosenman, R. H. Biological, psychological and social characteristics of men with different smoking habits. *Health Services Reports*, 1973, *88*, 834–843.

Jenkins, C. D., Zyzanski, S. J., & Rosenman, R. H. Risk of new myocardial infarction in middle-aged men with manifest coronary heart disease. *Circulation*, 1976, *53*, 342–347.

Jenkins, C. D., et al. Prediction of clinical coronary heart disease by a test for the coronary-prone behavior pattern. *New England Journal of Medicine*, 1974, *290*, 1271–1275.

Johannsen, W. J., et al. On accepting medical recommendations—Experiences with patients in a cardiac work classification unit. *Archives of Environmental Health*, 1966, *12*, 63–69.

Kahn, A. J. *Social policy and social services.* New York: Random House, 1973.

Kannel, W. B., & Dawber, T. R. Contributors to coronary risk implications for prevention and public health: The Framingham Study. *Heart and Lung*, 1972, *1*, 797–809.

Kannel, W. B., & Gordon, T. (Eds.). *The Framingham Study: An epidemiological investigation of cardiovascular disease* (Sections 1–32). Washington, D.C.: U.S. Department of Health, Education, and Welfare, 1977.

Kannel, W. B., Sorlie, P., & McNamara, P. M. Prognosis after initial myocardial infarction: the Framingham Study. *American Journal of Cardiology*, 1979, *44*, 53–59.

Kaplan, B. H. et al. Social supports and health. *Medical Care*, 1977, *5*, 47–58.

Kasl, S. Issues in patient adherence to health care regimens. *Journal of Human Stress*, 1975, *1*, 5–17.

Kasl, S., & Cobb, S. Health behavior, illness behavior, and sick role behavior. *Archives of Environmental Health*, 1966, *12*, 246–266.

Kegeles, S. S. Why people seek dental care: A test of a conceptual formulation. *Journal of Health and Human Behavior*, 1963, *4*, 166–173.

Kegeles, S. S. Attitudes and behavior of the public regarding cervical cytology: Current findings and new directions for research. *Journal of Chronic Diseases*, 1967, *20*, 911–922.

Kegeles, S. S. A field experimental attempt to change beliefs and behavior of women in an urban ghetto. *Journal of Health and Social Behavior*, 1969, *10*, 115–125.

Kendell, R. E. The classification of depressions: A review of contemporary confusion. In G. Burrows (Ed.), *Handbook of studies on depression*. New York: Excerpta Medica, 1977.

Kenigsberg, D., Zyzanski, S. J., Jenkins, C. D., et al. The coronary-prone behavior pattern in hospitalized patients with and without coronary heart disease. *Psychosomatic Medicine*, 1974, *36*, 344–351.

Kirscht, J. The health belief model and illness behavior. *Health Education Monographs*, 1974, *2*, 387–407.

Kitagawa, E. M., & Hauser, P. M. *Differential mortality in the United States: A study in socioeconomic epidemiology*. Cambridge, Mass.: Harvard University Press, 1973.

Klarman, H. F. Socioeconomic impact of heart disease. Second National Conference on Cardio-vascular Diseases, *The heart and circulation*, (Vol. 2). Washington, D.C.: Federation of American Societies for Experimental Biology, 1965, pp. 693–707.

Koslowsky, M., Croog, S. H., & La Voie, L. Perception of the etiology of illness: Causal attributions in a heart patient population. *Perceptual and Motor Skills*, 1978, *47*, 475–485.

Langner, T. S., & Michael, S. T. *Life stress and mental health*. Thomas A. C.

Rennie Series in Social Psychiatry (Vol. II). London: The Free Press of Glencoe, 1963.

Leighton, A. H. *My name is legion.* New York: Basic Books, Inc., 1959.

Ley, P., & Spelman, M. S. Communications in an outpatient setting. *British Journal of Social and Clinical Psychology*, 1965, *4*, 115–116.

Litman, T. J. The family as a basic unit in health and medical care: A social behavioral overview. *Social Science and Medicine*, 1974, *8*, 495–519.

Lowenthal, M. F. Some potentialities of a life-cycle approach to the study of retirement. In F. M. Carp (Ed.), *Retirement.* New York: Behavioral Publications, Inc., 1972, pp. 307–336.

Lowenthal, M. F. et al. *Four stages of life: A comparative study of women and men facing transitions.* San Francisco: Jossey-Bass, 1975.

Mann, G. V. Diet-heart: End of an era. *New England Journal of Medicine*, 1977, *296*, 644–650.

Marston, M. V. Compliance with medical regimens: A review of the literature. *Nursing Research*, 1970, *19*, 312–323.

Maas, H., & Kuypers, J. A. *From thirty to seventy: A forty year longitudinal study.* San Francisco: Jossey-Bass, 1974.

Mechanic, D. *Medical sociology.* New York: Free Press, 1978.

Medley, M. L. Satisfaction with life among persons sixty-five years and older: A causal model. *Journal of Gerontology*, 1976, *31*, 448–455.

Merton, R. K. *Social theory and social structure* (Rev. Ed.). New York: Free Press, 1957.

Mitchell, J. H. Compliance with medical regimens: An annotated bibliography. *Health Education Monographs*, 1974, *2*, 75–87.

Mushkin, S. J., and Collings, F. d'A. Economic costs of disease and injury. *Public Health Reports*, 1959, *74*, 795–809.

National Center for Health Statistics, *Inpatient utilization of short-stay hospitals by diagnosis: United States—1965*, Washington, D.C.: The Center, Series 13, No. 6, 1970.

National Center for Health Statistics, The national ambulatory medical care survey: 1975 summary, *Vital and health statistics*, Series 13, No. 33 (DHEW Pub. No. (PHS) 78–1784, Public Health Service). Washington, D.C.: U.S. Government Printing Office, January, 1978.

National Health Survey, *Prevalence of chronic circulatory conditions: United States, 1972*, Series 10, No. 94 (Publication No. (HRA) 75–1521).

Washington, D.C.: United States Department of Health, Education, and Welfare, September, 1974.

National Heart, Lung, and Blood Institute. *Report of the working group on heart disease epidemiology.* Bethesda, Md.: December, 1978.

Naughton, J., & Hellerstein, H. (Eds.). *Exercise testing and exercise training in coronary heart disease.* New York: Academic Press, 1973.

New York Heart Association, Criteria Committee, *Nomenclature and criteria for diagnosis of diseases of the heart and great vessels,* (7th ed.). Boston: Little, Brown and Company, 1973.

Osler, W. *Lectures on angina pectoris and allied states,* New York: D. Appleton and Company, 1892.

Palmore, E. (Ed.). *Normal aging: Reports from the Duke Longitudinal Study, 1955–1969.* Durham, N.C.: Duke University Press, 1970.

Palmore, E. (Ed.). *Normal aging II: Reports from the Duke Longitudinal Study, 1970–1973.* Durham, N.C.: Duke University Press, 1974.

Palmore, E., & Maddox, G. L. Sociological aspects of aging. In E. W. Busse & E. Pfeiffer (Eds.), *Behavior and adaptation in late life* (2nd Ed.). Boston: Little, Brown and Company, 1977, pp. 31–59.

Rae, J. B. The influence of the wives on the treatment outcome of alcoholics: A follow-up study of two years. *British Journal of Psychiatry,* 1972, *120,* 601–613.

Reeder, L. G. et al. Stress and cardiovascular health: An international cooperative study—II. The male population of a factory at Zurich. *Social Science and Medicine,* 1973, 7, 585–603.

Rice, D. P. *Economic costs of cardiovascular diseases and cancer, 1962.* (Health Economics Series No. 5, DHEW). Washington, D.C.: U.S. Government Printing Office, 1965.

Rice, D. P. *Estimating the cost of illness* (Health Economics Series No. 6). Washington, D.C.: U.S. Government Printing Office, 1966.

Riley, M. W., & Foner, A. (Eds.). *Aging and society: An inventory of research findings* (Vol. 1). New York: Russell Sage Foundation, 1968.

Rogot, E. Smoking and mortality among U.S. veterans. *Journal of Chronic Diseases,* 1974, *27,* 189–203.

Rosati, R. A., et al. A new information system for medical practice. *Archives of Internal Medicine,* 1975, *135,* 1017–1024.

Rosenman, R. H, & Friedman, M. Association of specific behavior pattern in women with blood and cardiovascular findings. *Circulation,* 1961, *24,* 1173–1184.

Rosenstock, I. M. What research in motivation suggests for public health. *American Journal of Public Health*, 1960, *50*, 295–302.

Rosenstock, I. M. The health belief model and preventive health behavior. *Health Education Monographs*, 1974, *2*, 354–386.

Rosenzweig, N. Some differences between elderly people who use community resources and those who do not. *Journal of the American Geriatrics Society*, 1975, *23*, 224–233.

Sackett, D., & Haynes, R. B. (Eds.). *Compliance with therapeutic regimens.* Baltimore: Johns Hopkins University Press, 1976.

Sanne, H. *Readaptation after myocardial infarction.* Monograph No. One. International Exchange of Information in Rehabilitation. World Rehabilitation Fund: New York, 1979.

Schwartz, D., et al. Medication errors made by elderly, chronically ill patients. *American Journal of Public Health*, 1962, *52*, 2018–2029.

Seigel, D. G., & Loncin, H. A critique of studies of long-term survivorship of patients with myocardial infarction. *American Journal of Public Health*, 1969, *58*, 1352.

Shanas, E. *Medical care among those aged 65 and over* (Research Series No. 16, Center for Health Administration Studies). Chicago: University of Chicago Press, 1960.

Shanas, E. Adjustment to retirement: Substitution or accommodation? In F. M. Carp (Ed.), *Retirement.* New York: Behavioral Publications, Inc., 1972, pp. 219–243.

Shapiro, S., et al. The H. I. P. study of incidence and prognosis of coronary heart disease, *Journal of Chronic Disease*, 1965, *18*, 527–558.

Shapiro, S., Weinblatt, E., & Frank, C. W. et al. Social factors in the prognosis of men following first myocardial infarction. *Milbank Memorial Fund Quarterly*, 1970, *48*, 37–50.

Shapiro, S., Weinblatt, E., & Frank, C. W. Return to work after first myocardial infarction. *Archives of Environmental Health*, 1972, *24*, 17–26.

Shekelle, R. B., Schoenberger, S. A., & Stamler, J. Correlates of the JAS Type A behavior pattern score. *Journal of Chronic Diseases*, 1976, *29*, 381–394.

Sheppard, H. L. Work and retirement. In R. H. Binstock & E. Shanas (Eds.), *Handbook of aging and the social sciences,* New York: Van Nostrand Reinhold Company, 1976, pp. 286–309.

Simon, A., et al. *Crisis and intervention: The elderly mental patient.* San Francisco: Jossey-Bass, 1970.

Skelton, M., & Dominian, J. Psychological stress in wives of patients with myocardial infarction. *British Medical Journal,* 1973, *2,* 101–103.

Smith, R. T., & Lilienfeld, A. L. *The Social Security Disability Program: An evaluation study* (Publication Number (SSA) 72–11801). Washington, D.C.: United States Department of Health, Education and Welfare, 1971.

Solon, J. A., et al. Linking young and old institutionalized people. *Public Health Reports,* 1977, *92,* 57–64.

Spreitzer, E., & Snyder, E. E. Correlates of life satisfaction among the aged. *Journal of Gerontology,* 1974, *29,* 454–458.

Streib, G. F. Morale of the retired. *Social Problems,* 1956, *3,* 270–276.

Sussman, M. B. The isolated nuclear family: Fact or fiction. *Social Problems,* 1959, *6,* 333–340.

Sussman, M. B. Readjustment and rehabilitation of patients. In J. Kosa et al. (Eds.), *Poverty and health: A sociological analysis.* Cambridge, Mass.: Harvard University Press, 1969.

Sussman, M. B. The family life of old people. In R. H. Binstock & E. Shanas (Eds.), *Handbook of aging and the social sciences.* New York: Van Nostrand Reinhold Company, 1976, pp. 218–248.

Taietz, P. Community complexity and knowledge of facilities. *Journal of Gerontology,* 1975, *30,* 357–362.

Task Force on Cardiac Rehabilitation, Report of the task force on cardiac rehabilitation, National Heart and Lung Institute (DHEW Publication No. (NIH) 75–750). Washington, D.C.: U.S. Government Printing Office, 1974.

Thiel, H. G., Parker, D., & Bruce, T. A. Stress factors and the risk of myocardial infarction. *Journal of Psychosomatic Research,* 1973, *17,* 43–57.

Thompson, E. L. Smoking education programs: 1960–1976. *American Journal of Public Health,* 1978, *68,* 250–257.

U.S. Department of Health, Education and Welfare, *Adult use of tobacco: 1970* (Public Health Service Publication No. (HSM) 73-8727). Washington D.C.: United States Government Printing Office, 1970.

U.S. Department of Health, Education and Welfare, *The health consequences of smoking—A report to the surgeon general: 1971* (Public Health Service Publication No. (HSM) 71–7513). Washington, D.C.: United States Government Printing Office, 1971.

U.S. Department of Health, Education and Welfare, Public Health Service, *Health: United States, 1978* (DHEW Pub. No. (PHS) 78–1232). Washington, D.C., U.S. Government Printing Office, 1978.

U.S. Department of Health, Education and Welfare, Public Health Service, Changes in cigarette smoking and current smoking practices among adults: United States, 1978 (DHEW Publication No. (PHS) 79–1250). *Advance data from vital and health statistics*, No. 52, September 19, 1979a.

U.S. Department of Health, Education and Welfare, *Smoking and health: A report of the surgeon general* (DHEW Publication No. (PHS) 79–50066). Washington, D.C.: Public Health Service, United States Government Printing Office, 1979b.

Villafana, C., & Mackbee, J. The value of continued follow-up in a preventive medicine program. *Industrial Medicine and Surgery*, 1971, *40*, 11.

Weinblatt, E., Shapiro, S., & Frank, C. W. Prognosis of women with newly diagnosed coronary heart disease—A comparison with course of disease among men. *American Journal of Public Health*, 1973, *63*, 577–593.

Weinblatt, E., et al. Relation of education to sudden death after myocardial infarction. *The New England Journal of Medicine*, 1978, *299*, 60–97.

Weintraub, M., et al. Compliance as a determinant of serum digoxin concentration. *Journal of the American Medical Association*, 1973, *224*, 481–485.

Weissman, M. M., & Paykel, E. S. *The depressed woman: A study of social relationships*. Chicago: University of Chicago Press, 1974.

Wenger, N. K., & Hellerstein H. K. (Eds.). *Rehabilitation of the coronary patient*. New York: Wiley and Sons, 1978.

White, P. D., et al. *Rehabilitation of the cardiovascular patient*. New York: McGraw-Hill, 1958.

AUTHOR INDEX

SUBJECT INDEX

Activity, level of patient, 51, 52
  and age, 56
  and depressive reaction, 193
  impact of illness upon, 102
  impairment of, 38, 51, 52
  See also Exercise; Physical activity,
    at work; Rest
Age of patients, 17, 43, 96, 250–252,
281, 287
  in analysis, 28, 29, 250
  and bed days reported, 53
  and cardiac morbidity and mortal-
    ity, 43, 44, 49, 50, 52, 53, 56, 62,
    140, 251
  and cigarette smoking, 147
  and compliance, 24, 132–134, 139–
    141, 251, 254
  and health services, use of, 23,
    114, 115
  and outcome, 28, 29, 220, 222,
    250–252
  and physician services, use of, 114,
    115, 251
  and retirement, 119, 251, 252
  and Social Security, use of, 118,
    119
  and support, patterns of, 26
  and symptoms reported, 50,
53

and Worker's Compensation, use
  of, 121–123
Aging, as characteristic of study
population, 18, 28, 29, 250
  and emotional status among heart
    patients, 25, 26
  and heart disease, adjustment to,
    250–252
  and quality of life, 27, 28
Alcohol consumption, physician
advice on, and patient compliance,
129, 130, 133, 134
Ambition, in factor analysis of
psychological self-ratings, 63, 181,
182, 187, 188, 211, 230, 232
American Cancer Society, 142
American Heart Association, 110,
142
Antecedent variables, and health status at Year 8, 53–70
  and outcome, 208–213, 218, 220–
    233
Anxiety, 19, 25, 48, 132, 196, 228,
264
  in wives of patients, 158, 159, 265
Armory of resources, classification
of, 209–212, 243–245
  elements in, 37, 75, 90, 125, 154,
    176, 255

as framework for analysis, 32–34,
202–213, 228, 232, 238
Base-line study, 17, 29, 30, 271–280
antecedent variables from, 202,
208–213, 218, 220–233, 247–252,
291, 292, 294, 295, 297–299
case distributions in, 274–280
cigarette smoking by patients and
wives, 25, 143–149
compliance of patients, 24, 25,
130–132, 134, 135, 137–139, 141,
254
depressive reaction of patients, 68,
192–197
family and social networks, 26, 27,
102, 159–164, 166, 261, 262
financial status of patients, 87, 90,
96–102, 257, 258
methodology, 29–32, 271–274,
288, 289
morbidity and mortality, 37, 38,
57, 67–70, 107, 108
psychological characteristics of patients and wives, 63, 177, 181–
186, 189
services, use of, 22, 106, 111, 255
work experience of patients, 22,
66, 78–90, 111, 256, 259
Bed days, reported by patients, 52,
53
Blue-collar workers (see Occupational
level)

Cancer, in patient population, 38
Cardiac rehabilitation unit, 110, 111,
255
Cash benefit programs, as resource,
97, 112, 113, 212, 244, 260, 261
Chest pain, reported by patients, 47,
48
Children, of patients, 155, 162
and etiology, patient perceptions
of, 165–167, 265, 266,
illness in, 161
impact of illness upon, 156–159,
265, 266

as resource, 167, 168, 170, 261,
262
Chiropractors, patient contact with,
108, 109
Clergy, patient contact with, 110,
111, 268
Clinics, patient use of, 106, 107
and age, 114, 115
Compliance, literature on, 23–25,
126, 131, 133, 134, 140, 142
measurement of, 126, 127
Compliance behavior, compared with
compliance orientation, 127, 128
smoking as example of, 126, 128,
142–149, 254
Compliance orientation, of patients,
125–142, 253–255
assessment of, 127, 128
and compliance behavior, 127, 128
correlates of, 132–135, 254, 255
definition of, 126, 127
over time, 130, 132, 134, 135, 254
and physician advice items, 129–
135, 253, 254
Compliance Orientation Index, 135–
142
classification by means of, 136, 139
correlates of, 138–142
definition of, 136
and information overload, 135,
136, 138, 139
over time, 137, 138, 141
Confidant, presence of, and outcome, 233, 235, 238, 249
and subjective stress, 198
Coronary personality, issues of, 62–
64, 176, 177, 179, 180, 182, 183,
186, 187, 189, 190, 211, 263, 264
Coronary-prone behavior pattern (see
Coronary personality, issues of)

Data collection, 29–32, 273, 274
Deaths (see Mortality)
Denial, 25, 68, 156, 157, 164, 266
Depression, and heart disease, 19,
25, 68, 191, 192, 265

Family, of patients, 154–173
  and etiology, 165–167, 265, 266
  illness in, 160, 161
  impact of illness upon, 27, 154–
    165, 265, 266, 270
  as resource, 26, 27, 96, 97, 154,
    167–173, 211, 213, 244, 249, 261,
    262, 265, 269, 270
  structure of, 155
  See also Kin and quasi-kin; Wives;
    Children
Finances, 90, 96–102
  costs of illness, 95, 96, 99–101, 258
  employment of wives, 102, 158,
    160, 258
  impact of illness upon, 87, 93, 96–
    102, 258, 259
  income, of patients, loss of, 87, 96,
    98, 99
  sources of, 96, 97
  marital disagreement regarding,
    162, 163
  See also Cash benefits, as resource;
    Income, level of patient
Financial assistance, patient receipt
  of, 96–98, 112, 113, 171–173, 260,
  261
Financial problems, patient perception of, 96, 101, 102, 258, 259
Framingham Heart Study, 21, 42
Friends, as resource (*see* Kin and
  quasi-kin, as resource)

Group therapist, patient contact with,
  110

Health, concern of patients about,
  102, 258, 259
Health behavior, difficulties in
  changing, 142, 257
Health Belief Model, 24, 147
Health Insurance Plan (H.I.P.), 21,
  42
Health outcome, 37–53, 247, 248
  and age, 43, 44, 49, 50, 52, 53, 56

  antecedents and correlates of, 53–
    70, 247, 248, 250
  assessment of, 38, 55, 56
  and depressive reaction, 68–70,
    247, 248, 264
  and health status in first year, 67–
    70
  and psychological characteristics of
    patients, 62–64
  and socioeconomic status, 57–62
  and work stress, 64–67
  See also Illness level; Physician
    ratings; Rehospitalization; Severe
    recurrences
Health policy, implications of study
  for, 159, 229, 243, 252, 267–270
Health services, patient use of (*see*
  Services)
Health status, of patients (*see* Health
  outcome; Illness level; Physician
  ratings; Rehospitalization; Severe
  recurrences)
Heart disease, as cause of death, 19,
  38–43, 248
  See also Mortality, in patient
    population
  disability due to, 19, 52
  in family of patient, 161
  as reason for rehospitalization, 38–
    43, 46, 248
  research on adjustment to, 18–28
  risk factors, 53–55, 64–68, 145,
    191, 259, 260, 263, 264
Hollingshead Index of Social Position, 104, 281, 287
Hospital, patient use of, 107, 108,
  110, 212
  See also Clinics; Rehospitalization,
    of patients

Illness, perceived gains from, as
  antecedent of outcome, 211, 223,
  225
  and depressive reaction, 192, 193
  as index of outcome, 206, 215–218

'ㅜ